Cytokines, Growth Mediators and Physical Activity in Children during Puberty

Medicine and Sport Science

Vol. 55

Cytokines, Growth Mediators and Physical Activity in Children during Puberty

Volume Editors

J. Jürimäe Tartu
A.P. Hills Brisbane
T. Jürimäe Tartu

29 figures, and 9 tables, 2010

KARGER

Basel · Freiburg · Paris · London · New York · Bangalore · Bangkok · Shanghai · Singapore · Tokyo · Sydney

Medicine and Sport Science
Founded 1968 by E. Jokl, Lexington, Ky.

Jaak Jürimäe, PhD
Institute of Sport Pedagogy and Coaching Sciences
University of Tartu
18 Ülikooli Street
Tartu 50090 (Estonia)

Andrew P. Hills, PhD
Institute of Health and Biomedical Innovation
Queensland University of Technology
60 Musk Avenue, Kelvin Grove
Brisbane, Queensland 4059 (Australia)

Toivo Jürimäe, PhD
Institute of Sport Pedagogy and Coaching Sciences
University of Tartu
18 Ülikooli Street
Tartu 50090 (Estonia)

Library of Congress Cataloging-in-Publication Data

Cytokines, growth mediators, and physical activity in children during puberty / volume editors, J. Jürimäe, A.P. Hills, T. Jürimäe.
p. ; cm. -- (Medicine and sport science, ISSN 0254-5020 ; v. 55)
Includes bibliographical references and indexes.
ISBN 978-3-8055-9558-2 (hard cover : alk. paper) -- ISBN 978-3-8055-9559-9 (e-ISBN)
1. Puberty. 2. Cytokines. 3. Growth factors. 4. Exercise--Physiological aspects. I. Jürimäe, Jaak. II. Hills, Andrew P. III. Jürimäe, T. IV. Series: Medicine and sport science ; v. 55. 0254-5020
[DNLM: 1. Puberty--physiology. 2. Adolescent Development--physiology. 3. Intercellular Signaling Peptides and Proteins. 4. Peptide Hormones--physiology. 5. Physical Exertion--physiology. W1 ME649Q v.55 2010 / WS 450]
QP84.4.C98 2010
612.6'61--dc22

2010029710

Bibliographic Indices. This publication is listed in bibliographic services, including Current Contents® and Index Medicus.

www.karger.com
Printed in Switzerland on acid-free and non-aging paper (ISO 9706) by Reinhardt Druck, Basel
ISSN 0254–5020
ISBN 978–3–8055–9558–2
e-ISBN 978–3–8055–9559–9

Contents

Preface

Over many centuries, scientists have been fascinated by the complexities of human growth and development and, accordingly, extensive research investigations have been undertaken. We understand, for example, that linear growth and sexual maturation are governed by the actions of the endocrine system, including the growth hormone (GH)-insulin-like growth factor 1 (IGF-1) axis, the hypothalamic-pituitary-gonadal (HPG) axis and thyroid hormone concentrations. While prepubertal growth is almost exclusively dependent on GH, IGF-1 and thyroid hormones, the marked acceleration in growth velocity during puberty is dependent on the interaction of the GH-IGF-1 and HPG axes with the continued permissive effect of thyroid hormones. A number of excellent monographs have addressed the role of the endocrine system in the growth and development of children and adolescents.

Somatic growth and maturation are also influenced by the nutritional status and level of physical activity of an individual. Growth and maturation are slowed during undernutrition, while chronic overnutrition may result in early maturation and increased growth velocity. The influence of nutritional status on linear growth and pubertal timing is also demonstrated by the fact that a critical amount of body fat is known to be essential for the onset of puberty. Similarly, the level of physical activity may have profound effects on children's health during pubertal development and influence the development of fat, muscle and bone tissue. These effects are mediated, at least partially, by the relationship between nutritional status, physical activity level, growth factors and also circulating inflammatory mediators/cytokines. These mediators are secreted from adipocyte, muscle and bone cells, and include, for example, leptin, interleukin-6 and osteocalcin, respectively. To date, the most extensively studied adipocytokine is leptin, which appears to be the molecular link between adequacy of energy stores, adipose tissue and the onset of puberty in children. The initiation of puberty has been linked to increased leptin and decreased ghrelin concentrations, while the recently discovered obestatin has been associated with obesity in childhood. The discovery of different inflammatory mediators/cytokines that contribute to the regulation of energy intake and energy expenditure is growing rapidly. For example, we have recently demonstrated that visfatin, a newly discovered marker of visceral adipose tissue, may have a metabolic role in adolescent male swimmers.

As an increasing proportion of children worldwide are involved in sport and physical activity, there is a need for more research on the exercise-related adaptation of adipose and bone tissue markers in young athletes. Increased participation of children and adolescents in competitive sport, especially when associated with inadequate caloric intake, exposes young athletes to numerous health risks including anorexia nervosa and reproductive dysfunction. The female athletic triad is characterized by late menarche, restrained eating behavior, and increased predisposition to stress fractures. We know that prolonged energy deficiency is related to alterations in body composition, including bone mineral density and bone turnover markers in adolescent athletes. Therefore, it is important to monitor pubertal athletes to better understand the influence of training loads on various hormonal markers that are responsible for growth and energy homeostasis. These hormonal markers also include different growth factors and circulating inflammatory mediators/cytokines.

To the best of our knowledge, no monographs to date have focused specifically on the complex relationship between inflammatory mediators/cytokines, growth factors, body composition, physical fitness and physical activity during puberty. In this book we focus on the latest research regarding mediators of growth and sexual maturation. Special emphasis has been given to the role of recently discovered inflammatory mediators/cytokines in the development of possible metabolic risk factors, in bone metabolism and other body composition parameters, in the development of possible menstrual irregularities and also in the adaptation to acute and chronic exercise. The 12 chapters comprising this monograph represent the latest information regarding the role of different inflammatory mediators/cytokines in the growth and pubertal development of children. Contributors include leading international researchers in this area who provide details of new developments regarding growth and development with particular relevance to researchers, students, pediatricians, coaches and other sport specialists.

Jaak Jürimäe, Tartu
Andrew P. Hills, Brisbane
Toivo Jürimäe, Tartu

Jürimäe J, Hills AP, Jürimäe T (eds): Cytokines, Growth Mediators and Physical Activity in Children during Puberty.
Med Sport Sci. Basel, Karger, 2010, vol 55, pp 1–13

An Overview of Physical Growth and Maturation

Andrew P. Hills · Nuala M. Byrne

Institute of Health and Biomedical Innovation, Queensland University of Technology, Brisbane, Queensland, Australia

Abstract

An understanding of physical growth and maturation is relevant to many disciplines, including exercise and sport science, anthropology, human biology, medicine, psychology and education. Growth and maturation is governed by a complex interaction between genetic and environmental factors. There is increasing evidence that physical activity plays an important role in normal growth, development, health and well-being of children and youth, however, caution is required in the activity setting so that growth and maturation is not jeopardised. To appreciate the impact of physical activity and/or exercise on growth and maturation, a thorough understanding of the general principles of auxology is useful. Following an introduction to terminology, an overview of physical growth and development is provided in the context of morphological changes. Detailed information is provided regarding individual variability in growth and development along with sexual dimorphism. A small degree of sexual dimorphism exists at birth however striking differences develop during the pubertal years. Sexual dimorphism in body composition is largely regulated by endocrine factors with critical roles played by growth hormone and gonadal steroids.

Introduction

Study of the pattern of growth in children and adolescents (auxology) has a long and rich history and is important across the biological continuum from conception to physical maturation. Accordingly, physical growth and maturation is relevant to many disciplines, including exercise and sport science, anthropology, human biology, medicine, psychology and education.

An appreciation of the concepts of growth, development and maturation is of particular importance in the context of children and adolescents who participate in sport and physical activity as exercise is one of many factors with the potential to influence growth and maturation [1, 2]. Changes in health and motor-related fitness are influenced by growth and maturation [2]; however, it is difficult to separate the specific

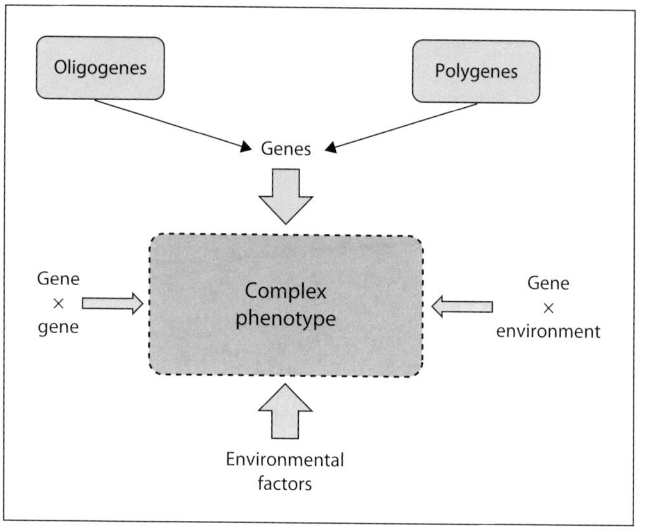

Fig. 1. Complex phenotypes – including obesity. Adapted from Comuzzie [10].

effects of physical activity on health and fitness from the growth and development process per se [3]. Despite increasing evidence to support the importance of physical activity to normal growth, development, health and well-being of children and youth [4–7], caution is required in the activity setting so that growth is not jeopardised [8].

Growth and maturation during infancy, childhood and adolescence are governed by genetic and environmental factors [9]. Comuzzie [10] suggests that the complex phenotype of obesity and related chronic conditions are the product of the action (as well as interaction) of multiple genes and environmental factors (fig. 1). Additionally, for all individuals, the environment exerts a strong influence on physical activity [11].

During the formative years, both nutrition and physical activity influence the growth and maturation of body fat, skeletal muscle tissue and bone [12]. Importantly, growth and maturation continues in times of limited physical activity [13]; however, appropriate nutrition is essential for optimal growth and development [2]. In short, when nutrition and physical activity during the growing years are appropriate, healthy patterns of physical maturation consistent with genetic potential may be expected. To understand the impact of physical activity and/or exercise on child growth and maturation, a thorough understanding of the general principles of auxology is important. The following section provides an overview of key terminology.

Terminology

In the context of physical growth, *growth* refers to an increase in physical size of the whole body or any of its component parts such as fat, muscle, and bone [9, 14].

Growth	Maturation	Development
Physical size	Skeletal	Social
Physique (shape or somatotype)	Neuromuscular	Emotional
Body composition	Sexual	Motor
Cardiovascular factors		
Self-concept, self-esteem, perceived readiness		

Fig. 2. Biopsychosocial matrix. Adapted from Malina et al. [18].

In contrast, *development* indicates an increase in skill and complexity of function, for example, neuromuscular control and motor skill. Development progresses as a function of growth, maturation and learning. Physical *maturation,* or level of physical development, can be defined as the distance one has travelled toward mature adult size and shape [15, 16]. In the growth and development context, maturation can also be viewed in terms of tempo and/or timing [14]. *Tempo* refers to the rate of progression of maturation whereas *timing* refers to the time at which specific maturity-related events occur, for example *peak height velocity* (PHV) and *menarche* (first menstruation) [17]. The term *morphology* is used to reference size and shape of the body.

Overview of Growth, Development and Maturation

The interactions between growth, development, and maturation govern many of the child's experiences during their first two decades of life [16]. Normal growth and development tracks in a consistent fashion but the major periods of physical growth are somewhat arbitrary in terms of chronological age. An appreciation of the gender and individual differences in the time course of physical growth and maturation is very useful from many perspectives, including for physical activity and sport.

Generally, growth and development are continuous and gradual processes however periods of more rapid growth are seen during infancy (the first year of life), the time of PHV, and puberty. There is also a predictable order in human development, for example, fundamental motor skills occur in the same sequence in all individuals, largely governed by the maturation of the central nervous system [2]. Individual differences in growth and development contribute to variability in the attainment of motor milestones and physical maturation. However, individual differences in a broader context are influenced by a complex interplay of biopsychosocial factors which are summarized in figure 2. It is important to acknowledge that the physical consequences of growth and development can be discussed in isolation but in reality a myriad of associated changes are occurring at the same time. For example, Malina [18] referred to a matrix of factors which contribute to individual differences in biological maturation which include variation in the timing and the tempo of the growth spurt and sexual maturation, plus psycho-social constructs such as self-concept, self-esteem, social status and socialization. Maturational changes in bone, muscle and fat are amongst the more important aspects of physical growth during adolescence as they alter height, weight and body proportions and define the gender differences in body composition. These issues will be discussed in more detail in the following sections.

Morphological Changes in Childhood and Adolescence

Size and shape of the human body is influenced by a combination of genetic and environmental factors. For example, tempo of growth, timing and rate of sexual development, skeletal maturation, dental development and adult stature are all significantly influenced by genetic factors with estimates of genetic transmissibility ranging from 41 to 71% [19, 20]. Tanner [19] claimed that the genetic control of the tempo of growth appears to be independent of that for body size and shape, and environmentally induced changes in tempo do not seem to significantly alter adult height or shape.

A range of environmental factors can modify one's genetic growth potential. For example, at birth, an infant's size is more dependent on maternal nutrition and intrauterine and placental factors than on genetic make-up [21]. Growth and development differences are also related to gender with sex-specific patterns seen in the tempo of growth, timing of the adolescent growth spurt, morphology, and age of skeletal maturity. Gender differences are evident from the fetal period and at birth females are 4–6 weeks more skeletally mature, a trend which continues across the balance of the growing years.

Growth velocity is slightly slower in females at birth with male neonates 1% longer and females slightly fatter [22]. Growth velocity is equivalent at approximately 7 months of age and is then somewhat faster in females until 4 years of age. Linear growth generally decelerates within the first 2 years of life and is relatively steady throughout childhood until the onset of the pubertal growth spurt [23]. Boys and girls grow at approximately the same rate, 5–6 cm/year and 2.5 kg/year [19]. Females on average enter puberty 2 years earlier than males but have a lower PHV (9 cm compared with 10.3 cm) and subsequent adult stature [24, 25]. Boys continue the pubertal growth spurt for approximately 1 year longer [23] with resultant increases in leg length, bone size and total bone mass.

Puberty is one of the most dynamic periods of growth and development and is characterized by rapid changes in morphology and composition, all of which are sexually dimorphic. During pubertal development, interactions between growth hormone (GH) and the sex steroid hormones are pronounced. In adolescent boys, rising concentrations of testosterone during puberty are pivotal in augmenting spontaneous secretion of GH and production of insulin-like growth factor 1 (IGF-1). According to Rogol et al. [21], testosterone's stimulation of pituitary GH secretion is short-lived and is only evident peri-pubertally. Both GH and IGF-1 concentrations decrease significantly in late puberty and early adulthood despite continued high concentrations of gonadal steroid hormones [26]. Estrogen in contrast, modulates GH secretory activity in a disparate manner; low doses of estrogen stimulate IGF-1 production through enhanced GH secretion, but higher doses inhibit IGF-1 production at the hepatic level [27].

Bogin [23] indicates that the so-called adrenarche results in a number of key changes including increased secretion of adrenal androgen hormones which contribute to a cascade of events: acceleration in height plus transient acceleration of bone maturation, development of secondary sexual characteristics and changes in fat distribution. The sex steroid hormones also play crucial roles in the accumulation, metabolism and distribution of adipose tissue [28]. For example, testosterone and estrogen facilitate fat deposition in the abdominal and gluteo-femoral regions, respectively, while testosterone is particularly important for the increase in lean mass that occurs during puberty, especially in boys [23]. Despite the most pronounced effects of the sex steroid hormones being seen during puberty, there is increasing evidence that exposure to these hormones in fetal life may have long-term implications for phenotype [29, 30].

The contrasting effects of the sex hormones during puberty are predominantly responsible for the larger skeletal size of the average male [29]. Estrogen has a key role in the development of bone mass but also helps conserve bone mass, suppress bone turnover, and maintain a balance between bone formation and resorption [31]. Testosterone reduces bone resorption and increases periosteal apposition of bone. The coordination of the pubertal growth spurt [31] by these hormones also includes the role of serum estrogen in the initiation and then completion of the growth spurt through closure of epiphyseal growth plates [31]. Testosterone also plays a role but not in the absence of estrogen [29].

The onset of puberty corresponds to a skeletal or biological age of approximately 11 years in girls and 13 years in boys [32]. On average, girls enter and complete each stage of puberty earlier than boys however even among healthy children, the timing and tempo of puberty varies widely. Maturational status during puberty is quantified on the basis of development of breasts and pubic hair in girls and pubic hair and genitalia in boys (readers are referred to Tanner [33] for details).

The adolescent growth spurt is one of the landmarks of puberty. Growth velocity slows immediately before a rapid acceleration during mid-puberty. In girls, the timing of the pubertal growth spurt is typically at Tanner breast stage 3 and does not reach the same magnitude as in boys. The average PHV of girls is 9 cm/year at age 12 years with a total gain in height of 25 cm across the pubertal growth period [34]. In contrast, the average PHV in boys is 10.3 cm/year and 2 years later than girls, coinciding with Tanner genital stage 4. In boys, an average total of 28 cm in height is gained across the growth period [25, 34].

Gender differences in the duration of pre-pubertal growth, plus greater PHV in boys, results in a greater average adult height difference of 13 cm [19] or ≈7% [35]. The gender difference in adult stature is largely the consequence of greater leg length in boys which also impacts body proportions [29]. After a period of decelerating height velocity, closure of major epiphyseal growth plates (which also follow a distinct sequence of maturation) limits further increase in height. This occurs at a mean skeletal age of 15 years in girls and 17 years in boys [19].

As for increases in height, significant weight gain also occurs during puberty. Approximately 50% of adult body weight is gained during adolescence with peak weight velocity (PWV) in boys occurring at approximately the same time as PHV, an average of 9 kg/year. In girls, PWV trails PHV by approximately 6 months and reaches 8.3 kg/year at approximately 12.5 years of age [19]. During the latter stages of puberty, rate of weight gain shows a similar pattern of deceleration as for height velocity.

Due to the wide individual variation in timing of the pubertal growth spurt, there is also a wide range of physiologic variations in normal growth. Individual variation in growth is further complicated by early, normal or late maturation. Early-maturing individuals generally have a larger adolescent growth spurt compared to later maturers [36]. Adult height is not necessarily affected as late maturers have a longer pre-pubertal growing period which is balanced by the more vigorous growth spurt of early maturers. Normal individual variability in maturational status may also be increased by alterations in energy intake and expenditure, for example restrictive diets and/or excessive physical activity [21] and influence the linear growth of children.

Secular Trends in Size and Shape

According to Tanner [37] the first textbook on human growth was written by Johann Augustin Stoeller in 1729. Temporal changes in height and weight, the so-called secular trend in growth and maturation, has resulted in a progressively earlier age of onset of puberty or menarche. These secular changes are related to a range of factors including improvements in socio-economic status, nutritional factors, and ethnicity [30].

There is general agreement that in recent decades, height and menarcheal age have stabilized in most Western countries, however, this finding has been complicated by reports of earlier age of breast development in girls. Demerath et al. [38] contend that earlier breast development could be the result of the higher prevalence of childhood obesity, not necessarily that obesity results in earlier progression through pubertal stages. It is important to remember that despite the widespread use of Tanner staging [33], methodological inconsistencies in the assessment of puberty may also account for differences in reported findings [39, 40].

Whilst not the focus of this chapter, it has been suggested that a significant proportion of the increase in adult height may be the result of changes in the first 2 years of life [30, 41]. Early life growth characteristics and body composition status have increasingly been linked with a subsequent risk of chronic disease.

Sexual Dimorphism in Body Composition

A cursory glance at the overall size and shape of pre-pubertal children suggests similarity between genders; however, there are significant sex differences in body composition before puberty. To date, the reasons for pre-pubertal sexual dimorphism are unknown [42]. When matched for age, weight, and height, pre-pubertal girls generally have higher total body fat and percentage body fat but lower fat-free mass [43, 44] plus total body bone mineral content [45, 46]. Pre-pubertal girls also commonly have greater trunk fat than boys [47, 48] although evidence is inconclusive [49, 50].

One of the hallmarks of pubertal growth and maturation is magnification of male-female differences in body composition. This includes changes in the relative proportions of water, muscle, fat, and bone which are all hormonally driven [29]. The large variability in maturational development among girls of the same chronological age means that hormonal and body composition changes during the pubertal period are best studied in relation to age at menarche rather than chronological age [33]. Increases in bone mineral content, muscle mass and deposition of body fat are governed by the sex hormones and GH. Changes in body fat distribution during this period, for example predisposition to central vs. peripheral, subcutaneous vs. visceral, and upper vs. lower body fat [21] contributes to the typical android and gynoid patterns of fat distribution of older male and female adolescents and adults, respectively [51]. Sexual dimorphism has also been described using the terms 'hourglass' to depict the female form and 'inverted triangle' for males characterized by broad shoulders and narrow waist [29].

By early adulthood there is marked dimorphism in total body composition with women having a greater mean percent body fat and relatively less lean mass. Using the body mass index (BMI), both sexes have relatively similar weight for height, however, the ratio of lean to fat is much greater in males [52]. It is important to highlight that the BMI is an inadequate index of body composition during growth. Typically, increases in BMI are attributed to greater fatness but age-related increases in BMI, particularly in boys, can be attributed to increments in lean mass rather than fat [53, 54].

Interestingly, sex differences in body composition are minimized at opposite ends of the body weight and disordered eating spectrum. For example, at one end of the spectrum restricted energy intake and/or increased energy expenditure impacts body shape by preventing post-pubertal tissue accretion while obesity at the other end decreases sexual dimorphism in shape and predisposes a more android fat distribution.

In boys, the significant increase in bone and muscle growth plus a concurrent reduction in limb fat is influenced by testosterone [19]. Maximal changes in these components of body composition in the upper extremity coincide with the time of PHV. In boys, the significant increase in lean body mass exceeds the total gain in weight because of the concomitant loss of adipose tissue. As height velocity declines, fat accumulation resumes in both sexes but is twice as rapid in girls [21]. In adulthood, males have approximately 150% of the lean body mass of the average female and twice the number of muscle cells [55].

The sex difference in bone mineral mass and skeletal size also becomes obvious during puberty [56, 57] at approximately 15–17 years of age and is influenced by both the longer pre-pubertal growth period of boys and the inhibitory effect of estrogen on periosteal apposition in girls [45]. There is a concomitant increase in muscular strength in males [58]. In adolescents who have completed normal pubertal growth and development, over 90% of peak skeletal mass is evident by 18 years of age [21]. In girls, approximately one-third of total bone mineral is accumulated in the 3 to 4 years following the onset of puberty [59, 60] such that at the start of adulthood, skeletal weight is ≈4 kg in men and 2.8 kg in women [61].

Impact of Obesity

The metabolic, hormonal and body composition changes during rapid pubertal growth can influence risk factors for chronic diseases such as type 2 diabetes. These dramatic physical growth and development changes increase adolescent requirements for energy, protein, vitamins and minerals. Therefore, nutrition is an important regulator of the tempo of human growth.

Obesity is commonly associated with taller stature in childhood and earlier pubertal development. In contrast, poor childhood nutrition delays the tempo of growth and pubertal onset [30]. Despite the fact that obese children (without endocrine abnormalities) are tall for their age, final adult height is consistent with their genetic background. On average, it has been estimated that obese children are 0.6 SD taller than normal-weight controls with a more advanced pubertal stage rating (0.4) on the Tanner scale [62].

The relationship between increased childhood weight gain, fat acquisition and earlier pubertal maturation has been explored over many years [63–65]. Girls with a relatively higher BMI are also more likely to have an earlier menarche [66]. Reasons for the differential in stature may include advanced skeletal age and both earlier adrenarche [67] and puberty [68]. Adrenarche usually precedes puberty by up to 2 years and is reflected by increased levels of the adrenal androgens dehydroepiandrosterone (DHEA) and dehydroepiandrosterone sulphate (DHEAS), independent of pituitary hypothalamic activation but partly controlled by adrenocorticotropic hormone (ACTH). Adrenarche is often more pronounced in obese children [30].

Evidence from a number of epidemiological studies indicates a relationship between earlier puberty in girls and increased BMI, the most commonly used indirect measure of obesity. Increased BMI is also correlated with the earlier attainment of other pubertal markers in girls including breast and pubic hair development. There is also increasing evidence that leptin has direct effects on gonadotropin secretion and may provide the link between body fat stores and the timing of puberty [66].

Physical Training and Growth

Over many years there has been interest in the impact of sports training on growth and development of children and adolescents. Certain sports, including female gymnastics [70] have received more attention however, relatively little consideration has been paid to the impact of growth and maturation per se in relation to exercise [17].

Roemmich et al. [71] contend that participation in sports where weight control is not required does not seem to affect pubertal timing or alter linear growth rate. The growth and maturation of athletes in weight control sports face the additional burden of a negative energy balance (energy expenditure greater than intake); however, it is uncommon for an energy deficit to be great enough to slow growth and maturation.

Marked undernutrition combined with heavy training and competition can suppress growth and maturation and delay pubertal development. Whether subsequent growth is disproportionate or not is hard to determine but the marked delay in the onset of estrogen action can permanently cause the skeleton to be undermineralized. In conclusion, most athletes continue to track along the centiles of their genetic potential. To define the mechanisms of growth and maturational delay one must longitudinally study children in weight-control sports.

It is logical to suggest that growth and maturation may influence the exercise and activity behaviors of children and adolescents, particularly when maturity-associated variation in size, proportions, body composition, and functional capacity are more pronounced [16]. In males, earlier growth and maturation is associated with greater gains in height, weight, weight-for-height, muscle mass and superior performance in many physical tasks [17]. Consequently, early maturing males have a distinct advantage in sport and physical activity, particularly when muscular strength, speed, and power are involved. Similarly, advanced maturation in females is associated with greater gains in height, weight, and weight-for-height. In contrast to males, gains in weight are predominantly associated with increased fat rather than muscle mass. Therefore, average and late-maturing females are advantaged in physical activity and exercise, particularly where endurance or weight bearing is involved.

Not surprisingly, body size and maturational status are strong predictors of selection and subsequent performance in a range of junior sports [16, 69]. In short, early-maturing males and normal or late-maturing females are over-represented in many competitive youth sports [14].

Conclusions and Future Research

Growth and development is characterized by significant changes in physical size and maturity and governed by complex interactions between genes and the environment. A comprehensive understanding of the temporal changes in growth and maturation, including normal individual variability and sexual dimorphism, is important in the context of children in sport and physical activity. However, we have a relatively poor understanding of the impact of growth and maturation per se in relation to exercise. Similarly, there are increasing challenges to face in relation to the epidemic of childhood obesity with implications for body composition and health status. More research is needed during the pre-natal and early post-natal stages of growth and development to better understand the role of maternal and infant nutrition and physical activity on subsequent health of children and youth.

References

1 Baxter-Jones A: Growth and maturation; in Armstrong N, van Mechelen W (eds): Paediatric Exercise Science and Medicine, ed 2, revised. Oxford, Oxford University Press, 2008, pp 157–168.

2 Hills AP, King NA, Armstrong T: The contribution of physical activity and sedentary behaviours to the growth and development of children and adolescents. Sports Med 2007;37:533–545.

3 Hills AP: Physical activity and movement in children: its consequences for growth and development. Asia Pac J Clin Nutr 1995;4:43–45.

4 Cordain L, Gotshall RW, Eaton SB, Eaton SB III: Physical activity, energy expenditure and fitness: an evolutionary perspective. Int J Sports Med 1998;19: 328–335.

5 Booth FW, Chakravarthy MV, Spangenburg EE: Exercise and gene expression: physiological regulation of the human genome through physical activity. J Physiol 2002;543(2):399–411.

6 Chakravarthy MV, Booth FW: Eating, exercise, and 'thrifty' genotypes: connecting the dots toward an evolutionary understanding of modern chronic diseases. J Appl Physiol 2004;96:3–10.

7 Caine D, Maffulli N: Epidemiology of children's individual sports injuries; in Caine DJ, Maffulli N (eds): Epidemiology of Pediatric Sports Injuries: Individual Sports. Med Sport Sci. Basel, Karger, 2005, vol 48, pp 1–7.

8 Kirk S, Scott BJ, Daniels SR: Pediatric obesity epidemic: treatment options. J Am Diet Assoc 2005; 105:S44–S51.

9 Cameron N, Demerath EW: Growth, maturation and the development of obesity; in Johnston FE, Foster GD (eds): Obesity, growth and development. London, Smith-Gordon & Company, 2001, pp 37–55.

10 Comuzzie AG: The genetic contribution to human obesity: the dissection of a complex phenotype; in Johnston FE, Foster GD (eds): Obesity, Growth and Development. London, Smith-Gordon & Company, 2001, pp 21–36.

11 Dollman J, Norton K, Norton L: Evidence for secular trends in children's physical activity behaviour. Br J Sports Med 2005;39:892–897.

12 Meredith CN, Dwyer JT: Nutrition and exercise: effects on adolescent health. Annu Rev Public Health 1991;12:309–333.

13 Malina RM: Growth and maturation: do regular physical activity and training for sport have a significant influence?; in Armstrong N, van Mechelen W (eds): Paediatric Exercise Science and Medicine. Oxford, Oxford University Press, 2000, pp 95–106.
14 Malina RM: The young athlete: Biological growth and maturation in a biocultural context; in Smoll FL, Smith RE (eds): Children and Youth in Sports: A Biopsychosocial Perspective, ed 2. Dubuque, Kendall Hunt, 2002, pp 261–292.
15 Baxter-Jones ADG, Eisenmann JC, Sherar LB: Controlling for maturation in pediatric exercise science. Pediatr Exerc Sci 2005;17:18–30.
16 Malina RM, Bouchard C, Bar-Or O: Growth, Maturation, and Physical Activity, ed 2, revised. Champaign, Human Kinetics, 2004.
17 Cumming SP, Standage M, Gillison FB, Dompier TP, Malina RM: Biological maturity status, body size, and exercise behaviour in British youth: a pilot study. J Sports Sci 2009;27:677–686.
18 Malina RM: Childhood and adolescent obesity: selected issues and implications; in Johnston FE, Foster GD (eds): Obesity, Growth and Development. London, Smith-Gordon & Company, 2001, pp 1–20.
19 Tanner JM: Fetus into Man: Physical Growth from Conception to Maturity. Cambridge, Harvard University Press, 1989.
20 Sinclair D: Human Growth after Birth. London, Oxford University Press, 1978.
21 Rogol AD, Clark PA, Roemmich JN: Growth and pubertal development in children and adolescents: effects of diet and physical activity. Am J Clin Nutr 2000;72(suppl):521S–528S.
22 Rodriguez G, Samper MP, Olivares JL, Ventura P, Moreno LA, Perez-Gonzalez JM: Skin-fold measurements at birth: sex and anthropometric influence. Arch Dis Child 2005;90:F273–F275.
23 Bogin B: Patterns of Human Growth. Cambridge, Cambridge University Press, 1999.
24 Marshall WA, Tanner JM: Variations in patterns of pubertal changes in girls. Arch Dis Child 1969;44: 291–303.
25 Marshall WA, Tanner JM: Variations in patterns of pubertal changes in boys. Arch Dis Child 1970;45: 13–23.
26 Martha PM Jr, Rogol AD, Veldhuis JD, Kerrigan JR, Goodman DW, Blizzard RM: Alterations in the pulsatile properties of circulating growth hormone concentrations during puberty in boys. J Clin Endocrinol Metab 1989;69:563–570.
27 Ho KY, Evans WS, Blizzard RM, Veldhuis JD, Merriam GR, Samojlik E, Furlanetto R, Rogol AD, Kaiser DL, Thorner MO: Effects of age and sex on the 24-hour profile of growth hormone secretion in man: importance of endogenous estradiol concentrations. J Clin Endocrinol Metab 1987;64:51–58.
28 Norgan NG: The beneficial effects of body fat and adipose tissue in humans. Int J Obes 1997;21:738–746.
29 Wells JCK: Sexual dimorphism of body composition. Best Pract Res Clin Endocrinol Metabol 2007; 21:415–430.
30 Dunger DB, Ahmed ML, Ong KK: Effects of obesity on growth and puberty. Best Pract Res Clin Endocrinol Metabol 2005;19:375–390.
31 Riggs BL, Khosla S, Melton LJ: Sex steroids and the construction and conservation of the adult skeleton. Endocr Rev 2002;23:279–302.
32 Tanner JM, Whitehouse RH, Marshall WA, Carter BS: Prediction of adult height, bone age, and occurrence of menarche, at age 4 to 16 with allowance for mid-parental height. Arch Dis Child 1975;50:14–26.
33 Tanner JM: Growth at Adolescence. Oxford, Blackwell Scientific, 1962.
34 Kelch RP, Beitins IZ: Adolescent sexual development; in Kappy MS, Blizzard RM, Migeon CJ (eds): The Diagnosis and Treatment of Endocrine Disorders in Childhood and Adolescence, ed 4. Springfield, Thomas, 1994, pp 193–234.
35 Gustafsson A, Lindenfors P: Human size evolution: no evolutionary allometric relationship between male and female stature. J Hum Evol 2004;47:253–266.
36 Tanner JM, Whitehouse RH, Takaishi M: Standards from birth to maturity for height, weight, height velocity, and weight velocity: British children, 1965. Part I. Arch Dis Child 1966;41:454–471.
37 Tanner JM: A short walk in the garden of auxological delights; in Johnston ZB, Eveleth PB (eds): Human Growth in Context. London, Smith-Gordon Co Ltd, 1999, pp 1–14.
38 Demerath EW, Li J, Sun SS, Chumlea WC, Remsberg KE, Czerwinski SA, Towne B, Siervogel RM: Fifty-year trends in serial body mass index during adolescence in girls: the Fels Longitudinal Study. Am J Clin Nutr 2004;80:441–446.
39 Reiter EO, Lee PA: Have the onset and tempo of puberty changed? Arch Pediatr Adolesc Med 2001; 155:988–989.
40 Herman-Giddens ME, Kaplowitz PB, Wasserman R: Navigating the recent articles on girls' puberty in pediatrics: what do we know and where do we go from here? Pediatrics 2004;113:911–917.

41 Cole TJ: The secular trend in human physical growth: a biological view. Econ Hum Biol 2003;1: 161–168.
42 Garnett SP, Högler W, Blades B, Baur LA, Peat J, Lee J, Cowell CT: Relation between hormones and body composition, including bone, in pre-pubertal children. Am J Clin Nutr 2004;80:966–972.
43 Taylor RW,Gold E, Manning P, Goulding A: Gender differences in body fat content are present well before puberty. Int J Obes 1997;21:1082–1084.
44 Mast M, Kortzinger I, Konig E, Muller MJ: Gender differences in fat mass of 5–7-year old children. Int J Obes 1998;22:878–884.
45 van der Sluis IM, de Ridder MAJ, Boot AM, Krenning EP, de Muinck Keizer-Schrama SMPF: Reference data for bone density and body composition measured with dual energy X-ray absorptiometry in white children and young adults. Arch Dis Child 2002;87:341–347.
46 Horlick M, Thornton J, Wang J, Levine LS, Fedun B, Pierson RN Jr: Bone mineral in prepubertal children: gender and ethnicity. J Bone Miner Res 2000; 15:1393–1397.
47 Arfai K, Pitukcheewanont PD, Goran MI, Tavare CJ, Heller L, Gilsanz V: Bone, muscle, and fat: sex-related differences in pre-pubertal children. Radiology 2002;224:338–344.
48 Herd SL, Gower BA, Dashti N, Goran MI: Body fat, fat distribution and serum lipids, lipoproteins and apolipoproteins in African-American and Caucasian-American prepubertal children. Int J Obes 2001;25:198–204.
49 He Q, Horlick M, Thornton J, Wang J, Pierson RN, Heshka S, Gallagher D: Sex and race differences in fat distribution among Asian, African-American, and Caucasian prepubertal children. J Clin Endocrinol Metab 2002;87:2164–2170.
50 Cowell CT, Briody J, Lloyd-Jones S, Smith C, Moore B, Howman-Giles R: Fat distribution in children and adolescents – the influence of sex and hormones. Horm Res 1997;48(suppl 5):93–100.
51 Johnston FE: Developmental aspects of fat patterning; in Hernandez M, Argente J (eds): Human Growth: Basic and Clinical Aspects. Amsterdam, Elsevier, 1992, pp 217–226.
52 Wells JCK: The evolution of human fatness and susceptibility to obesity: an ethological approach. Biol Rev 2006;81:183–205.
53 Wells JCK: A Hattori chart analysis of body mass index in infants and children. Int J Obes 2000;24: 325–329.
54 Maynard LM, Wisemandle W, Roche AF, Chumlea WC, Guo SS, Siervogel RM: Childhood body composition in relation to body mass index. Pediatrics 2001;107:344–350.
55 Cheek DB: Body composition, hormones, nutrition and adolescent growth; in Grumbach MM, Grave GD, Mayer FE (eds): Control of the Onset of Puberty. New York, Wiley, 1974, pp 424–447.
56 Maynard LM, Guo SS, Chumlea WC, Roche AF, Wisemandle WA, Zeller CM, Towne B, Siervogel RM: Total-body and regional bone mineral content and areal bone mineral density in children aged 8–18 y: the Fels Longitudinal Study. Am J Clin Nutr 1998;68:1111–1117.
57 Nguyen TV, Maynard LM, Towne B, Roche AF, Wisemandle W, Li J, Guo SS, Chumlea WC, Siervogel RM: Sex differences in bone mass acquisition during growth: the Fels Longitudinal Study. J Clin Densitom 2001;4:147–157.
58 Schoenau E, Neu CM, Rauch F, et al: The development of bone strength at the proximal radius during childhood and adolescence. J Clin Endocrinol Metabol 2001;6:613–618.
59 Bonjour J, Theintz G, Buchs B, Slosman D, Rizzoli R: Critical years and stages of puberty for spinal and femoral bone mass accumulation during adolescence. J Clin Endocrinol Metab 1991;73:555–563.
60 Slemenda CW, Reister TK, Hui SL, Miller JZ, Christian JC, Johnston CC: Influence on skeletal mineralization in children and adolescents: evidence for varying effects of sexual maturation and physical activity. J Pediatr 1994;125:201–207.
61 Malina RM: Regional body composition: age, sex and ethnic variation; in Roche AF, Heysnfield SB, Lohman TG (eds): Human Body Composition. Champaign, Human Kinetics, 1996.
62 Wells JC, Fewtrell MS, Williams JE, et al: Body composition in normal weight, overweight and obese children: matched case-control analyses of total and regional tissue masses, and body composition trends in relation to relative weight. Int J Obes 2006;30: 1506–1513.
63 Garn SM, Haskell JA: Fat and growth during childhood. Science 1959;130:1711–1712.
64 Garn SM, LaVelle M, Pilkington JJ: Comparisons of fatness in premenarcheal and postmenarcheal girls of the same age. J Pediatr 1983;102:328–331.
65 Adair LS, Gordon-Larsen P: Maturational timing and overweight prevalence in US adolescent girls. Am J Public Health 2001;91:642–644.
66 Kaplowitz PB: Link between body fat and the timing of puberty. Pediatrics 2008;121(suppl 3): S208–S217.
67 Neville KA, Walker JL: Precocious pubarche is associated with SGA, prematurity, weight gain, and obesity. Arch Dis Child 2005;90:258–261.

68 Kaplowitz PB, Slora EJ, Wasserman RC, et al: Earlier onset of puberty in girls: relation to increased body mass index and race. Pediatrics 2001;108:347–353.
69 Cumming SP, Eisenmann JC, Smoll FL, Smith RE, Malina RM: Body size and perceptions of coaching behaviors by adolescent female athletes. Psychol Sport Exerc 2005;6:693–705.
70 Rogol AD, Roemmich JN, Clark PA: Growth at puberty. J Adolesc Health 2002;31(6 suppl):192–200.
71 Roemmich JN, Richmond RJ, Rogol AD: Consequences of sport training during puberty. J Endocrinol Invest 2001;24:708–715.

Prof. Andrew P. Hills, PhD
Institute of Health and Biomedical Innovation, Queensland University of Technology
60 Musk Avenue, Kelvin Grove
Queensland 4059 (Australia)
Tel. +61 7 3138 6087, Fax +61 7 3138 6030, E-Mail a.hills@qut.edu.au

Jürimäe J, Hills AP, Jürimäe T (eds): Cytokines, Growth Mediators and Physical Activity in Children during Puberty.
Med Sport Sci. Basel, Karger, 2010, vol 55, pp 14–31

Role of Various Cytokines and Growth Factors in Pubertal Development

Krista Casazza · Lynae J. Hanks · Jessica A. Alvarez

Department of Nutrition Sciences, University of Alabama at Birmingham, Birmingham, Ala., USA

Abstract

Historical data suggest that body composition is intricately involved in pubertal development. Progression through puberty is dependent on the interaction between the growth hormone-insulin-like growth factor-1 (GH-IGF-1) axis, reproductive and metabolic hormones as well as pro- and anti-inflammatory cytokines which induce alterations in feedback mechanisms and therefore mediate body composition and growth. Simultaneous increases in GH and IGF-1, and the concomitant changes in the hormonal milieu (i.e. reproductive hormones, testosterone and estrogen, and insulin) are the major contributors to anabolic effects seen throughout the pubertal transition, and are affected by various factors including (but not limited to) energy status and body composition. Orexigenic agents (i.e. ghrelin and leptin) also play a role at the level of the hypothalamus affecting not only energy intake, but also pubertal onset and progression. Effects of cytokines, many of which may be considered catabolic, extend beyond their traditionally viewed role involving the immune system, accompanying reproductive maturity further regulating aspects of energy and bone metabolism. As such, the signal(s) initiating the hypothalamic response that triggers puberty is likely reliant on a number of neural, metabolic and endocrine networks, all of which are at least partially influenced by pubertal growth factors, and act independently, antagonistically and/or synergistically to regulate anabolic pathways, therefore modifying body composition trajectory and growth during adolescence.

Introduction

Adolescence is a period of rapid growth and development culminating in full reproductive maturation. Major anabolic regulators induce marked changes in physiology and metabolism driving the pubertal transition and subsequent changes in body composition. Normal adolescent development is largely regulated through the growth hormone-insulin-like growth factor-1 (GH-IGF-1) axis [1]. However, there are also additional factors related to sexual maturation as well as metabolic signals that influence body composition or contribute to body tissue partitioning during puberty via direct or indirect effects on growth hormone (GH) and/or insulin-like growth factor-1 (IGF-1) expression and abundance. For example, reproductive hormones have effects on fuel utilization and partitioning of resources as well as impact the secretion of GH and/or IGF-1 [2–4]. Metabolic cues from hormones such as insulin and ghrelin also enhance growth during puberty [5, 6]. Additionally, various cytokines are involved in body composition changes during the pubertal transition, though not all are anabolic [7]. Further, chronic inflammation, a state observed in obesity, may result in alterations in the expression and or function of growth factors that influence body composition trajectories and impact long-term metabolic health [8, 9]. The purpose of the present review is to evaluate some interesting findings related to various growth factors and cytokines in pubertal development (fig. 1).

Anabolic Effects of Growth Factors during the Pubertal Transition

The pubertal transition is characterized by interplay between the somatotrophic and gonadotrophic hormonal axes, combining mitogenic and metabolic actions. The increases in GH during the pubertal transition influence somatic growth, substrate metabolism and a growth spurt, leading to dramatic changes in body composition. Further, GH induces local IGF-1 production in the ovaries and testes, activating the hypothalamic-pituitary-gonadal (HPG) axis, playing a major role in the regulation of pubertal growth [9–11] The simultaneous increases in GH and IGF-1 concentration and the concomitant changes in the hormonal milieu suggest regulatory interactions in the secretion and action of these factors (fig. 1).

Growth Hormone

The primary hormone responsible for the pubertal growth spurt is GH. The growth-promoting effects of GH in puberty are realized across a number of tissues: propeptides from collagen fibers stimulate bone and non-bone collagen synthesis; increase protein synthesis and muscle mass through sarcomere hyperplasia; increase resting energy expenditure (REE), fat oxidation and hepatic gluconeogenesis; and decrease fat deposition, hepatic glucose uptake, and insulin sensitivity [11]. Puberty is delayed in GH-deficient children indicating direct regulation of GH in pubertal growth [3]. During puberty, GH secretion is markedly increased resulting in peak levels of IGF-1 [11]. Negative feedback control of GH secretion is mediated by its own secretion as well as IGF-1 by the direct action on the somatotroph and on hypothalamic growth hormone releasing hormone (GHRH) and somatostatin neurons. Other regulators of GH include metabolic cues of insulin, glucose, nonesterified fatty acids, pro-inflammatory cytokines, as well as certain amino acids. Additionally, partitioning of resources (i.e. deposition of fuel as fat, lean or bone) influence and are influenced by GH levels.

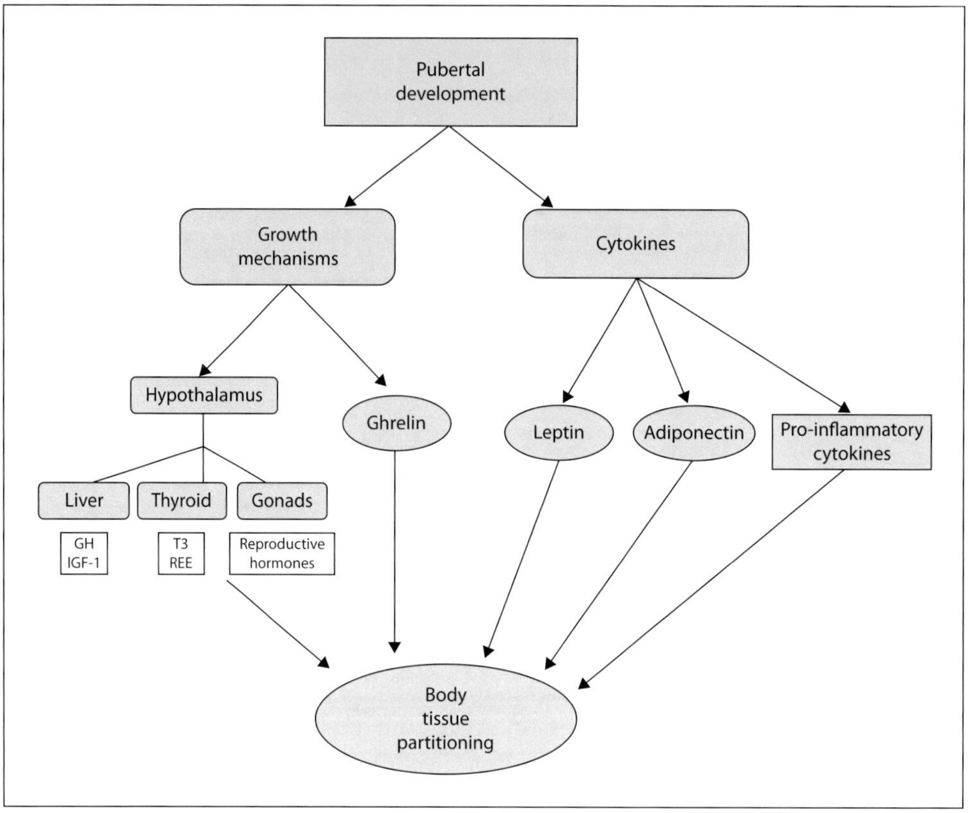

Fig. 1. Mitogenic and metabolic interplay between the somatotrophic and gonadotrophic hormonal axes during pubertal transition. Simultaneous changes in growth mechanisms and cytokines initiate concomitant changes influencing regulatory mechanisms associated with body composition.

Energy status (i.e. available fuel for tissue partitioning) contributes to alterations in GH levels. Undernourished adolescents have higher GH levels, as opposed to those with high adiposity [12]. In adolescents with anorexia nervosa, GH levels have been shown to be higher when compared with healthy controls. Further, low levels of GH are frequently reported in adolescents with obesity, as the condition is a potent negative regulator of GH. Data also suggest that lower GH levels found in obese adolescents relate to higher trunk fat and lipid levels as compared with their normal-weight peers [13]. In addition, disorders resulting in GH deficiency (i.e. acromegaly) predispose to abdominal fat accumulation and unfavorable lipid profiles. Interestingly, abdominal obesity, associated with an increase in pro-inflammatory cytokines, may be a primary contributor to the decline in GH status associated with excess adipose tissue. Together, these data suggest alterations in GH levels may lead to aberrations in body composition affecting regional fat deposition and adverse metabolic profiles. As such, the implications of fat mass accumulation during puberty may have profound

Table 1. Growth factors and their function during pubertal development

Growth factor	Secreted from	Main function in puberty
GH	anterior pituitary	↑ IGF-1 release
		↑ bone growth
		(↑ chondrogenesis, ↑ Ca absorption, epiphyseal growth plate widening)
		↑ RMR
		↑ lean mass
		↓ fat mass
		↓ hepatic glucose output
		↑ lipolysis
IGF-1	liver	↑ cell growth and multiplication (↑ DNA synthesis)
		↑ RMR
		↑ lean mass
		↑ bone
		↑ chondrogenesis
		↓ programmed cell death
Testosterone	testes	sexual maturity
Estrogen	ovaries	sexual maturity
Thyroid hormone	thyroid	metabolic rate
Insulin	pancreas	↑ glucose uptake in the liver, muscle, and fat tissue ↑ glycogen in the liver and muscle ↓ fat as an energy source.
Ghrelin	stomach	energy balance

effects on hormonal feedback mechanisms which may manifest in adverse body tissue partitioning and impaired future metabolic health (table 1).

Insulin-Like Growth Factor-1

The IGF axis is a system of growth mediators, receptors and binding proteins. Almost every cell in the human body is affected by IGF-1, the major component of the IGF

Table 2. Ranges of select growth factors during the pubertal transition

Tanner stage	IGF-1 ng/ml[a]		Testosterone ng/dl[b]		Estradiol pg/ml[b]		Insulin µU/ml[c]		Leptin µg/l[d]		Adiponectin µg/ml[h]	
	M	F	M	F	M	F	M	F	M	F	M	F
I	63–279	49–342	<7–20	<7–20	U–13	U–20	9.7 ± 4.9	10.1 ± 5.8	0.65–3.04	1.23–5.12	12.4–16.2	10.9–14.2
II	75–240	115–428	8–66	<7–47	U–16	U–24	12.5 ± 6.9	14.0 ± 6.5	0.91–5.28	1.51–5.44	10.6–13.3	11.5–15.7
III	94–765	145–760	26–800	17–75	U–26	U–60	15.4 ± 9.1	14.0 ± 7.6	0.48–3.29	1.93–7.51	9.1–11.9	11.2–14.3
IV	192–861	244–787	85–1,200	20–75	U–38	15–85	11.6 ± 2.4	12.7 ± 6.4	0.38–1.64	2.67–7.23	8.7–10.7	11.9–14.6
V	171–422	143–859	300–950	12–60	10–40	15–350	8.6 ± 4.1	11.7 ± 4.8	0.34–1.44	3.57–10.89	8.4–11.5	10.0–12.6
Adults (19 years+)	53–527[b]	53–442[b]	240–950	8–60	10–40	15–350[e] <10[f]	2.6–25[b]	2.6–25[b]	0.7–5.3[b,g]	3.3–18.3[b,g]		

M = Males; F = females; U = undetectable. [a] Central 95% ranges reported by Elmlinger et al. (2004). [b] Mayo Clinic Medical Laboratories Reference Values (www.mayomedicallaboratories.com). [c] Values are mean ± SD reported by Gower et al. (2003). [d] Values are ± 1 SD from medians reported by Blum et al. [66]. [e] Premenopausal women. [f] Postmenopausal women. [g] Based on a lean adult. [h] Adiponectin 95% CI reported by Kettaneh et al. [67].

axis postnatally [14]. IGF-1 has been associated with numerous biological processes including cell cycle regulation, differentiation, proliferation and apoptosis and acts both independently and in concert with GH directly promoting growth in the pubertal transition. The cell proliferative and anti-apoptotic effects may be promoted through direct interactions with other growth factors or indirect associations with steroid hormones and integrins [14]. IGF-1 also regulates peripheral neuroactive signaling for normal brain function, activates the expression of adrenal enzymes and interacts with reproductive hormones. The liver is the principal source of circulating IGF-1 with hepatic production stimulated by GH secretion (as well as nutritional factors). Generation and activity of IGF-1 are insulin dependent such that depressed insulin inhibits the IGF-1 system [15]. The majority of the IGFs in the circulation exist in a complex with respective binding proteins. Bound IGF-1 (~90% bound to IGF-binding protein-1 and -3; IGFBP-1 and IGFBP-3) accounts for nearly all of the circulating levels, with less than 1% free IGF-1 in circulation [16]. Pubertal circulating IGF-1 concentrations are approximately two to three times greater than during adulthood and increase with pubertal status (table 2) [2, 16, 17]. The molar ratio between IGF-1 and IGFBP-3 is a reflection of free, biologically active IGF-1 levels. Further, the ratio increases in puberty, suggesting a differential regulation of IGF-1 and IGFBP-3 [18].

Because of the differential impact of sex through varied reproductive hormone levels and timing of maturation, the pubertal influence on IGF-1 varies accordingly. Although there is a reversal in sexual dimorphism upon reproductive maturation, pre-pubertal girls have higher IGF-1 than do males [19]. Likewise, during puberty, IGF-1 concentrations are consistently higher in girls than boys, although there is a positive relationship between age and IGF-1 in boys [17]. These results are in agreement with the observation that girls experience peak height velocity, along with elevation of serum IGF-1 earlier than in boys. Since IGFBP-3 binds the majority of the IGFs, it is also of interest to note that girls have significantly higher levels of IGFBP-3 than boys throughout puberty [16].

As previously discussed, GH levels are decreased among individuals with obesity. Correspondingly, adolescent obesity has been associated with profound perturbations in the IGF system in both the basal state and in response to postprandial insulin changes [20]. Despite suppressed GH concentrations, however, the pubertal growth spurt of adolescents with obesity is not altered [20], and IGF-1 levels are not affected by body mass index (BMI) [16]. The apparent lack of variation in IGF-1 levels between normal and overweight adolescents may exist due to a protective mechanism of other growth factors. It has been hypothesized that leptin signaling in children with obesity may substitute for GH in terms of IGF-1 synthesis as an activator signal transducer and activator of transcription 5b (Stat5b), which is in the same family of transcription factors of IGF-1 [21]. Given the substantial role of the HPG axis in body composition trajectory during adolescence, small changes in IGF-1 concentration could have huge repercussions for a wide range of basic physiological and metabolic functions that influence growth and development and its relationship with health.

Reproductive Hormones

There is a positive association between GH, IGF-1 and reproductive hormones during puberty that significantly influences body tissue partitioning. Although reproductive hormones act directly on the growth plate independent of GH, a vast majority of sex-related differences in growth and development are likely to be mediated by the contribution of the reproductive hormones to changes in the GH-IGF-1 axis [4, 5]. Since GH secretion is increased by a similar magnitude in girls and boys during puberty, the interaction of the reproductive hormones and GH-IGF-1 is likely a major contributor of pubertal growth and development outcomes, as well as sexual dimorphism in body composition changes.

Testosterone is a potent stimulator of somatic tissue growth, particularly in terms of lean tissue [22]. Testosterone is involved in a positive feedback loop and both GH and testosterone are necessary for optimal anabolism [4, 5]. It has been shown that administration of exogenous testosterone leads to significant increases in GH and growth velocity [23]. However, testosterone did not appear to have independent effects that augment the IGF-1 response; therefore, testosterone alone may not have contributed anabolic effects. The independent and combined effects of testosterone was studied by Gibney et al. [24] in which IGF-1 was enhanced by testosterone in response to GH, yet IGF-1 concentrations were unchanged with testosterone alone. GH alone, on the other hand, stimulated REE and fat oxidation, and these changes were amplified with the co-administration of testosterone. These results indicate that the metabolic action of GH on anabolic body composition changes is enhanced by testosterone, with reduced independent effects of either hormone and that IGF-1 levels are indirectly impacted by the interaction of GH and testosterone. Reference values for testosterone concentrations are provided in table 2 by Tanner stage.

The anabolic effects of estrogen may be realized via indirect effects involved in pubertal onset initiation. Proximity to puberty results in marked alterations in hormonal activity initiated due to the dramatic stimulation of the HPG axis [5]. In females, the HPG axis is activated upon GH and IGF-1 stimulation of luteinizing hormone-releasing hormone (LHRH), leading to maturation and function of the ovary and resulting in both sexual maturation and a growth spurt. Estrogen has growth-enhancing effects through augmentation of chondrocyte proliferation at the growth plate [3]. Similarly, in boys, estrogen levels are positively associated with growth velocity prior to peak height. Unlike the effects of testosterone, once pubertal onset has ensued, both estrogen and estrogen-like compounds attenuate GH action, thus reducing IGF-1 levels [3, 25]. Further, estrogen concentration is negatively associated with growth velocity after peak height attainment [26]. It is uncertain if augmentation due to contribution of GH to chondrocyte proliferation may be mediating estrogen-enhancing growth since estrogen itself has major, sometimes opposing, effects on epiphyseal chondrocyte growth [25]. No evidence exists to clarify interdependent roles between estrogen and GH at the cellular level of the growth plate. Reference values for circulating estradiol are provided in table 2 by Tanner stage.

Estrogen regulates the metabolic effects of GH at the level of secretion and also at the level of GH signaling [25]. The estrogen-mediated reduction in GH signaling and subsequent IGF-1 production is due to inhibition of the GH receptor. Estrogen inhibits hepatic IGF-1 production in a dose-dependent manner, and at the cellular level inhibits GH signaling in a concentration-dependent manner. Interestingly, the negative regulation of the GH receptor by estrogen is induced by increased expression of suppressors of cytokine signaling (SOCS) proteins [25]. Therefore, though reproductive hormones may not be strictly anabolic per se, but influence the catabolic effects of pro-inflammatory cytokines (fig. 2). In females, estradiol is thought to be protective against inflammation in adulthood, however, the effects are unclear during developmental years.

Testosterone	Estradiol	SHBG
–IL6	–IL6	+IL6
+CRP	+CRP	–CRP
+TNFα	+TNFα	–TNFα
+Adiponectin	–Adiponectin	+Adiponectin
+/–Resistin	+Resistin	+/–Resistin
+Ghrelin	–Ghrelin	+/–Ghrelin
+/–Visfatin	+/–Visfatin	+/–Visfatin
–Leptin	+Leptin	+/–Leptin

Fig. 2. Relationships between testosterone (in males), estradiol (in females) and SHBG (both males and females) and cytokines during puberty.

Insulin

Insulin is an anabolic agent or a growth-promoting hormone. Circulating insulin concentration therefore plays a direct role in growth. A transient insulin-resistant state occurs during normal pubertal development with immediate presence at the beginning of puberty, a peak at mid-puberty in both sexes, and a decline to near pre-pubertal levels by early adulthood [27]. Characteristic of insulin resistance, during puberty, fasting insulin concentrations and plasma insulin responses to oral and intravenous glucose are higher than during earlier childhood and adulthood (table 2) [27]. The decrease in insulin sensitivity and subsequent elevated insulin concentrations during puberty likely contribute to the accelerated growth that occurs at this time [28].

The transient insulin resistance that occurs during puberty may be an important contributor to reproductive maturation and the timing of pubertal onset [28]. It has been proposed that the degree of insulin sensitivity (and resultant changes in the GH-IGF-1 axis due to amount of circulating insulin) may act as an important metabolic signal involved in the maturational changes of human adrenals at the time of adrenarche [28]. However, a sexual dimorphism may exist. Girls are known to have higher insulin resistance than boys, possibly relating to differences in adiposity between the sexes [29]. Potau et al. [30] found no association between insulin resistance and boys with pronounced adrenarche and precocious puberty. Further data from Guercio et al. [2] support the hypothesis that, in boys, neither the GH-IGF-1 axis nor insulin sensitivity is involved in adrenarche. However, in girls it was found that with premature adrenarche there was a deregulation of the insulin-IGF-1 system implying a role in the pathophysiology [31, 32]. Additionally, Guercio et al. [2] found a significant decrease of insulin sensitivity in normal pre-pubertal girls and during transition from late pre-puberty to early puberty. Nonetheless, the combination of rising GH, secretion of endogenous reproductive hormones, and rising insulin levels, in turn contributing to the alterations in IGF-1 secretion and production, may all contribute to and synergistically enhance growth during the pubertal period in both males and females (table 3).

Table 3. Summary of growth factor changes during puberty and metabolic effects

Growth factor	Pubertal changes	Obesity influences	Pubertal onset	Bone development
GH	↑	↓		+
IGF-1	↑	↓		+
Testosterone	↑		+	+
Estrogen	↑	↑	+	+
Progesterone	↑	↑	+	+
DHEAS	↑	↓	+	+
Thyroid hormone	↑	↓		+
Insulin	↑	↑	+	+
Ghrelin	↑	↓	+	+

Ghrelin

Ghrelin, an orexigenic agent, acts on the hypothalamus to increase food intake. It is increased in the fasted state and decreased in the fed state [33]. Ghrelin was initially identified and named due to its ability to elicit GH secretion [34]. The anabolic effect of ghrelin may be direct or mediated by GH production. As a potent stimulant of GH release, ghrelin also promotes lipolysis, gluconeogenesis and insulin secretion. Additionally, ghrelin is involved in cell proliferation [35]. Although identified as a signal of energy homeostasis, the effect of ghrelin on a variety of other systems continues to be identified.

During childhood, the effect of ghrelin level on appetite is not defined. Although it is well known that appetite and food intake during puberty are increased during puberty, it occurs despite decreasing ghrelin levels. This may be indicative of heightened sensitivity to the appetite-stimulative effects of the hormone during this period [36]. Recently, ghrelin has been hypothesized to provide another link between energy homeostasis, body composition and pubertal development through action on the hypothalamus [35]. There, ghrelin stimulates secretion of gonadotropin-releasing hormone (GnRH), which in turn, stimulates the pituitary production and secretion of the gonadotropins required for pubertal onset. Ghrelin concentrations decrease from the prepubertal to pubertal stage in both males and females [36]. For example, Whatmore et al. [36] report a decrease in ghrelin from 119–470 pg/ml in prepubertal boys to 88–304 pg/ml in pubertal boys and a decrease from 103–359 to 60–493 pg/ml in prepubertal and pubertal girls, respectively. However, the mechanisms linking ghrelin to pubertal onset as well as the physiological relevance of ghrelin to changes in body composition during puberty are not fully understood. It has been reported that ghrelin is inversely associated with BMI and percent fat in children and adolescents, and obese children and adolescents have lower total ghrelin than their normal weight counterparts [37]. However, weight loss in the obese subjects was not associated with significant changes in ghrelin concentrations, nor was it associated with insulin or the homeostatic model assessment of insulin resistance (HOMA-IR) after weight loss. Ghrelin may also influence bone metabolism. In vitro experiments show that ghrelin increases osteoblast proliferation [38]. In adolescent females, there was a positive association between ghrelin concentration and lumbar spine bone mineral apparent density, as well as hip bone mineral density [13] independent of relevant body composition and hormonal confounders, such as fat mass, estradiol and GH. Ghrelin, however, was not significantly associated with markers of bone turnover, thus the bone-forming effects of ghrelin may be mediated through other growth factors. Further, it has been reported that ghrelin dose-dependently inhibits cytokine mRNA expression. Although it is clear that the role of ghrelin extends beyond a satiety hormone, the extent to which ghrelin is involved in reproductive function, metabolism and growth has only recently been investigated.

Effects of Cytokines during the Pubertal Transition

Cytokines, although more commonly known for their effects on the immune system, are involved in various regulatory aspects of energy and bone metabolism [7, 9, 39, 40]. Cytokines are released by various cell types, such as adipocytes, macrophages, myocytes, and osteocytes; with those secreted by adipocytes typically referred to as adipocytokines. Cytokine/adipocytokine concentrations fluctuate and play a significant role during puberty, particularly in the regulation of energy intake, bone mass accrual and pubertal onset [6, 9, 40]. Although complex, it is clear that the intricate interactions among pro- and anti-inflammatory cytokines allow for a balance between body tissues during growth (table 4). The following sections discuss changes in specific cytokine/adipocytokine concentrations that occur during adolescence and their role in pubertal development.

Leptin

Leptin is an adipose-derived, anorexigenic factor involved in the hypothalamic regulation of satiety, body weight and energy expenditure. Due to its involvement in energy expenditure and subsequent regulation of body stores, leptin's role in pubertal growth and development is becoming increasingly more evident. In adolescents, as in adult populations, leptin increases with increasing adiposity [41], particularly in the

Table 4. Summary of cytokine changes during puberty and metabolic effects

Cytokine	Pubertal changes	Obesity influences	Pubertal onset	Bone development
IL-6	↓	↑		±
TNF-α		↑		–
Leptin	↑ (girls), ↓ (boys)	↑	+	±
Adiponectin	↓ (boys)	↓		–
Resistin	↑ / ↓ / Ø[a]	Ø / ↑		–[b]
Visfatin	↑ / ↓ / Ø[a]	↑		Ø[b]

↓ = Decrease; ↑ = increase; Ø = no change or no effect; + = promote; – = inhibit; [a] Longitudinal studies not available. [b] Has not been studied in adolescents.

subcutaneous department. Leptin also plays a key role in reproductive functioning and has been suggested to be a link between energy reserves and neuro-endocrine mechanisms in the pathway for reproductive maturity. However, whether there is a permissive effect of leptin on initiation of puberty and/or if pubertal onset is influenced directly by leptin or indirectly by body composition changes related to leptin, is not entirely clear.

The suggestion of leptin as a permissive factor in pubertal progression was first reported by Suter et al. [42] in which the effects of leptin on the stimulation of the GH-IGF-1 axis and pubertal initiation were observed in primates. More recently, the majority of studies have centered on the effects of leptin on regulation of GnRH, thus allowing for the pituitary secretion of gonadotropins necessary for pubertal onset [35]. Not only do GnRH neurons in the hypothalamus express leptin receptors, but the pulsatility of gonadotropin release by GnRH is stimulated by leptin [43]. Further, elevations in leptin levels may contribute to the activation of the HPG axis and may also lead to activation of the GH-IGF axis resulting in positive feedback to the HPG axis [35]. Circulating leptin is inversely associated with age at menarche, and due to the peak in leptin concentrations at pubertal onset, leptin has also been hypothesized to be the metabolic trigger for the initiation of puberty in males [43]. In prepubertal girls and boys, leptin concentration increases slowly with age-related fat mass increases. However, with increasing proximity to puberty, a sexual dimorphism in leptin concentrations becomes apparent [44, 45], in which leptin peaks at Tanner stage 5 in females and it peaks at Tanner stage 2 and decreases throughout pubertal progression in males (table 2). This supports the notion of a stimulatory effect of estrogen on leptin levels in females and a suppressive effect of testosterone on leptin levels in males [44]. The sexual dimorphism, as well as changes in circulating leptin occurring during adolescence, have been suggested to reflect a direct effect of adiposity on reproductive hormones [41].

Leptin may also play a role in the regulation of bone formation [46], although available evidence is equivocal. Leptin has been shown to inhibit osteoclast production and promote chondrocyte formation in vitro [46]. In human studies, among girls followed through the pubertal transition, leptin was found to be positively associated with change in bone area [47]. However, animal models suggest that leptin functioning through neural pathways is inhibitory to bone formation, whereas peripheral leptin effects promote bone formation [46]. Additionally, the influence of leptin on bone regulation may be influenced by stage in the life cycle and therefore its role in bone metabolism is not entirely clear.

Adiponectin

Unlike many of the other adipocytokines, adiponectin is expressed and secreted exclusively by adipose tissue [48]. This cytokine is commonly acknowledged for its potential insulin-sensitizing, anti-inflammatory, and anti-atherogenic effects. Adiponectin in pediatric populations and its relationship with insulin resistance and other metabolic risk factors have recently been extensively reviewed [49]. In brief, adiponectin concentrations generally decrease with increasing adiposity in adolescents, and in adolescents is generally positively associated with insulin sensitivity, independent of adiposity.

Circulating adiponectin concentrations are influenced by pubertal development, although changes are sex-specific [41]. Adiponectin concentrations do not change during puberty in females; however, concentrations decrease during puberty in males, specifically at mid-puberty, resulting in lower adiponectin concentrations in adolescent males than females. The decreased concentrations in males likely reflect direct inhibitory effects of androgens on adiponectin [49]. Given its relationship with insulin sensitivity, decreases in adiponectin may mediate the transient decrease in insulin sensitivity observed in males during adolescence; however, other factors may be involved in pubertal insulin resistance in girls and remain to be elucidated [50]. Adiponectin may have further roles in the regulation of bone metabolism which also are yet to be elucidated.

Pro-Inflammatory Cytokines

In addition to GH-inhibiting effects, during normal skeletal growth, pro-inflammatory cytokines play an integral role in the regulation of bone turnover. These cytokines are known promoters of osteoclast differentiation and its bone resorptive actions [51]. The source of many of these osteoclastogenic cytokines are osteoblasts.

Tumor Necrosis Factor-α

Tumor necrosis factor-α (TNF-α) is a pro-inflammatory cytokine produced by numerous cell types, including adipose tissue. It exerts numerous metabolic effects including appetite suppression, catabolism, suppression of insulin signaling, and promotion of other inflammatory cytokines and adipokines, with levels increasing as adiposity increases. It is a known bone resorptive agent as evidenced in vitro [52], in animal experiments [53], and in disease states characterized by chronic inflammation [54]. It is also a promoter of osteoclast formation (osteoclastogenesis), directly stimulating osteoclast progenitor differentiation and inducing osteoblast secretion of other pro-bone resorptive cytokines [36].

Polymorphisms of TNF-α have been suggested to play a role in bone size determination in adolescents [55]. In healthy female Caucasian adolescents, carriers of an A allele of the TNF-α gene had significantly greater lumbar spine bone area than those without, and this polymorphism was an independent predictor of lumbar spine bone area. Plasma TNF-α, although not significantly different among the genotypes, was also a positive independent predictor of lumbar spine bone area. The association between plasma TNF-α and lumbar spine bone area seems contradictory, however it may indicate greater bone turnover and formation in subjects with higher circulating TNF-α levels. Alternatively, greater circulating TNF-α may reflect less binding to receptors necessary for TNF-α-induced osteoclast differentiation. Indeed, genetic variation in the TNF-receptor 2 gene have been shown to be associated with lower bone mineral density [55].

Interleukin-6

Interleukin-6 (IL-6), derived primarily from adipose tissue and its related cytokines, have multiple functions including promotion of osteoclast activity [51]. It is positively associated with adiposity in adolescents, with obese adolescents experiencing chronic low-grade inflammation [56]. Concentrations of IL-6 significantly decrease during mid-to-late puberty [41], reflecting the need for reduced osteoclast activity to promote maximal bone growth. Production of IL-6 is inhibited by both androgens and estrogen, explaining the inverse association between circulating IL-6 and the reproductive hormones in adolescents [41].

Resistin

Resistin is an adipose-derived pro-inflammatory cytokine hypothesized to induce insulin resistance, and to be a possible link between obesity and diabetes [57]. Several studies have shown equivocal results regarding the relationship of resistin with obesity status in children and adolescents [37, 41], although a recent study in a large Chinese cohort did find children and adolescents with obesity to have significantly greater resistin concentrations than children with normal weight; adiposity measures were significantly associated with resistin in the pubertal adolescents only and no relationship was observed in the pre-pubertal group [58]. As such, the changes in resistin concentrations during puberty are not clear, as two additional studies found no differences in resistin between pre-pubertal and pubertal stages [37, 41] and another observed a positive association between resistin and reproductive maturation [59]. In general, studies in children and adolescents have shown girls to have greater resistin concentrations than boys [37, 58]. The gender differences in resistin concentrations may be mediated by differences in reproductive hormones, although the relationship has not been consistent among studies [41, 59]. Longitudinal studies investigating changes in resistin that occur with changes in pubertal development, including body composition, fat distribution, and reproductive hormone concentrations, are required for further elucidation of this relationship.

Despite the study differences in the relationships of resistin to adiposity and pubertal development, most studies in adolescents show that resistin is not associated with indices of insulin resistance, including HOMA-IR, fasting insulin and adiponectin concentrations, suggesting that resistin does not mediate insulin action in adolescents [37, 58, 59]. Direct measures of insulin action have not been investigated in relation to resistin in adolescents and should, thus, be considered for future research. In addition to adipose tissue, resistin is expressed by osteocytes and may play a regulatory role in bone homeostasis, as indicated in vitro, and by its inverse association with lumbar spine bone mineral density in Korean adult males [60]. Resistin has not been investigated in adolescents in relation to bone metabolism.

Visfatin

Visfatin, a recently discovered pro-inflammatory cytokine expressed in high levels by visceral adipose tissue [61], is hypothesized to play a role in mediating insulin activities. It is also considered a pro-inflammatory cytokine, due to its expression in numerous cells of the immune system and is induced by pro-inflammatory cytokines, such as IL-6 and TNF-α, and it can, likewise, induce the expression of these pro inflammatory cytokines [8]. Circulating visfatin concentrations in adolescents have been assessed in a small number of cross sectional studies; however, specific changes that occur during puberty have not been investigated. As with resistin, studies show conflicting results regarding the association of visfatin with age. Age has been shown to be positively associated with visfatin in Japanese children with obesity aged 5–15 years [62], negatively associated with visfatin in Chinese children with obesity aged 11–18 years [63], and have no significant relationship with visfatin in Austrian children with obesity aged 11–16 years [64]. Longitudinal studies in adolescents are required to determine if visfatin concentration is associated with pubertal development.

All studies to date have reported significantly higher visfatin concentrations in children and adolescents with obesity compared to those with normal weight [62, 64]. In addition, adolescent studies are consistent in that sex differences in visfatin concentrations have not been observed and that visfatin is not significantly associated with indices of glucose and insulin metabolism [62, 63]. Whether visfatin plays a role in bone metabolism has not been extensively investigated, although it was not significantly associated with bone mineral density in Chinese adult males [65]. The influence of visfatin on bone metabolism in adolescents has not been investigated.

Conclusions

The pubertal transition is a critical period for growth and development, particularly in terms of body tissue partitioning and metabolism. Progression through puberty is significantly associated with increases in GH, IGF-1 and reproductive hormone concentrations. The physiological adaptations to hormonal fluctuations, particularly upon pubertal onset, induce tissue hyperplasia and influence an inflammatory response. Between the sexes, striking differences in body composition and height emerge despite lack of significant differences in GH output. This implies an indirect stimulation of growth involving interplay between two systems representing a modulatory effect in which reproductive hormones attenuate and/or augment the accretion of GH.

Although the pubertal transition is known to be involved in the stimulation of anabolic growth factors, a concomitant release of cytokines, many of which may be considered catabolic, also accompanies reproductive maturity. During chronic inflammation as observed in obesity, inflammatory cytokines may induce further cytokine expression resulting in inhibition of GH and adverse effects on growth. It has been suggested that alterations in growth factor concentrations during pubertal development represent sensitivity for the programming of adult body habitus and health.

Growth and development during adolescence is complex, and is influenced by a number of pathways. The trigger of pubertal onset has been identified as increased hypothalamic release of GnRH, although the many factors leading up to this event have not been fully elucidated. The enigma is likely due to a variety of changes occurring simultaneously which vary based on several components, such as reproductive hormones, cytokines and other growth factors. The simultaneous body composition changes during pubertal development make the independent relationship between growth factors, cytokines and reproductive hormone concentrations as well as the catabolic versus anabolic effects on tissue partitioning, difficult to tease apart. Taken together, these factors act independently, antagonistically and/or synergistically to influence anabolic pathways, thereby modifying body composition trajectories during adolescence.

References

1 Hull KL, Harvey S: Growth hormone: a reproductive endocrine-paracrine regulator? Rev Reprod 2000;5:175–182.

2 Guercio G, Rivarola MA, Chaler E, Maceiras M, Belgorosky A: Relationship between the growth hormone/insulin-like growth factor-I axis, insulin sensitivity, and adrenal androgens in normal prepubertal and pubertal girls. J Clin Endocrinol Metab 2003;88:1389–1393.

3 Leung KC, Johannsson G, Leong GM, Ho KK: Estrogen regulation of growth hormone action. Endocr Rev 2004;25:693–721.

4 Meinhardt UJ, Ho KK: Modulation of growth hormone action by sex steroids. Clin Endocrinol (Oxf) 2006;65:413–422.

5 Meinhardt UJ, Ho KK: Regulation of growth hormone action by gonadal steroids. Endocrinol Metab Clin North Am 2007;36:57–73.

6 Tena-Sempere M: Roles of ghrelin and leptin in the control of reproductive function. Neuroendocrinology 2007;86:229–241.

7 McCann SM, Kimura M, Karanth S, Yu WH, Mastronardi CA, Rettori V: The mechanism of action of cytokines to control the release of hypothalamic and pituitary hormones in infection. Ann NY Acad Sci 2000;917:4–18.

8 Dedoussis GV, Kapiri A, Samara A, et al: Visfatin: the link between inflammation and childhood obesity. Diabetes Care 2009;32:e71.

9 MacRae VE, Wong SC, Farquharson C, Ahmed SF: Cytokine actions in growth disorders associated with pediatric chronic inflammatory diseases (review). Int J Mol Med 2006;18:1011–1018.

10 Belgorosky A, Baquedano MS, Guercio G, Rivarola MA: Expression of the IGF and the aromatase/estrogen receptor systems in human adrenal tissues from early infancy to late puberty: implications for the development of adrenarche. Rev Endocr Metab Disord 2009;10:51–61.

11 Robson H, Siebler T, Shalet SM, Williams GR: Interactions between GH, IGF-I, glucocorticoids, and thyroid hormones during skeletal growth. Pediatr Res 2002;52:137–147.

12 Misra M, Bredella MA, Tsai P, Mendes N, Miller KK, Klibanski A: Lower growth hormone and higher cortisol are associated with greater visceral adiposity, intramyocellular lipids, and insulin resistance in overweight girls. Am J Physiol Endocrinol Metab 2008;295:E385–E392.

13 Misra M, Miller KK, Almazan C, Worley M, Herzog DB, Klibanski A: Hormonal determinants of regional body composition in adolescent girls with anorexia nervosa and controls. J Clin Endocrinol Metab 2005;90:2580–2587.

14 Lin CM, Huang YL, Lin ZY: Influence of gender on serum growth hormone, insulin-like growth factor-I and its binding protein-3 during aging. Yonsei Med J 2009;50:407–413.

15 Lopez-Bermejo A, Khosravi J, Fernandez-Real JM, et al: Insulin resistance is associated with increased serum concentration of IGF-binding protein-related protein 1 (IGFBP-rP1/MAC25). Diabetes 2006;55:2333–2339.

16 Juul A, Dalgaard P, Blum WF, et al: Serum levels of insulin-like growth factor (IGF)-binding protein-3 (IGFBP-3) in healthy infants, children, and adolescents: the relation to IGF-I, IGF-II, IGFBP-1, IGFBP-2, age, sex, body mass index, and pubertal maturation. J Clin Endocrinol Metab 1995;80:2534–2542.

17 Lofqvist C, Andersson E, Gelander L, et al: Reference values for insulin-like growth factor-binding protein-3 (IGFBP-3) and the ratio of insulin-like growth factor-I to IGFBP-3 throughout childhood and adolescence. J Clin Endocrinol Metab 2005;90:1420–1427.

18 Kaplan RC, McGinn AP, Pollak MN, et al: Association of total insulin-like growth factor-I, insulin-like growth factor binding protein-1 (IGFBP-1), and IGFBP-3 levels with incident coronary events and ischemic stroke. J Clin Endocrinol Metab 2007;92:1319–1325.

19 Ong KK, Emmett P, Northstone K, et al: Infancy weight gain predicts childhood body fat and age at menarche in girls. J Clin Endocrinol Metab 2009;94:1527–1532.

20 Attia N, Tamborlane WV, Heptulla R, et al: The metabolic syndrome and insulin-like growth factor I regulation in adolescent obesity. J Clin Endocrinol Metab 1998;83:1467–1471.

21 Woelfle JF, Harz K, Roth C: Modulation of circulating IGF-I and IGFBP-3 levels by hormonal regulators of energy homeostasis in obese children. Exp Clin Endocrinol Diabetes 2007;115:17–23.

22 Bhasin S, Woodhouse L, Casaburi R, et al: Testosterone dose-response relationships in healthy young men. Am J Physiol Endocrinol Metab 2001;281:E1172–E1181.

23 Gibney J, Wolthers T, Johannsson G, Umpleby AM, Ho KK: Growth hormone and testosterone interact positively to enhance protein and energy metabolism in hypopituitary men. Am J Physiol Endocrinol Metab 2005;289:E266–E271.

24 Gibney J, Healy ML, Stolinski M, et al: Effect of growth hormone (GH) on glycerol and free fatty acid metabolism during exhaustive exercise in GH-deficient adults. J Clin Endocrinol Metab 2003;88:1792–1797.

25 Wolthers T, Hoffman DM, Nugent AG, Duncan MW, Umpleby M, Ho KK: Oral estrogen antagonizes the metabolic actions of growth hormone in growth hormone-deficient women. Am J Physiol Endocrinol Metab 2001;281:E1191–E1196.

26 Klein NA, Battaglia DE, Miller PB, Soules MR: Circulating levels of growth hormone, insulin-like growth factor-I and growth hormone binding protein in normal women of advanced reproductive age. Clin Endocrinol (Oxf) 1996;44:285–292.

27 Smith CP, Archibald HR, Thomas JM, et al: Basal and stimulated insulin levels rise with advancing puberty. Clin Endocrinol (Oxf) 1988;28:7–14.

28 Lee JM: Insulin resistance in children and adolescents. Rev Endocr Metab Disord 2006;7:141–147.

29 Moran A, Jacobs DR Jr, Steinberger J, et al: Insulin resistance during puberty: results from clamp studies in 357 children. Diabetes 1999;48:2039–2044.

30 Potau N, Ibanez L, Sentis M, Carrascosa A: Sexual dimorphism in the maturation of the pituitary-gonadal axis, assessed by GnRH agonist challenge. Eur J Endocrinol 1999;141:27–34.

31 Dunaif A: Insulin resistance and the polycystic ovary syndrome: mechanism and implications for pathogenesis. Endocr Rev 1997;18:774–800.

32 Ibanez L, Potau N, De ZF: Endocrinology and metabolism after premature pubarche in girls. Acta Paediatr Suppl 1999;88:73–77.

33 Cummings DE, Purnell JQ, Frayo RS, Schmidova K, Wisse BE, Weigle DS: A preprandial rise in plasma ghrelin levels suggests a role in meal initiation in humans. Diabetes 2001;50:1714–1719.

34 Kojima M, Hosoda H, Date Y, Nakazato M, Matsuo H, Kangawa K: Ghrelin is a growth-hormone-releasing acylated peptide from stomach. Nature 1999; 402:656–60.

35 Budak E, Fernandez SM, Bellver J, Cervero A, Simon C, Pellicer A: Interactions of the hormones leptin, ghrelin, adiponectin, resistin, and PYY3–36 with the reproductive system. Fertil Steril 2006;85: 1563–1581.

36 Whatmore AJ, Hall CM, Jones J, Westwood M, Clayton PE: Ghrelin concentrations in healthy children and adolescents. Clin Endocrinol (Oxf) 2003; 59:649–654.

37 Reinehr T: Obesity and thyroid function. Mol Cell Endocrinol 2010;316:165–171.

38 Maccarinelli G, Sibilia V, Torsello A, et al: Ghrelin regulates proliferation and differentiation of osteoblastic cells. J Endocrinol 2005;184:249–256.

39 Frost RA, Lang CH: Alteration of somatotropic function by proinflammatory cytokines. J Anim Sci 2004;82(E-suppl):E100–E109.

40 Pass C, MacRae VE, Ahmed SF, Farquharson C: Inflammatory cytokines and the GH/IGF-I axis: novel actions on bone growth. Cell Biochem Funct 2009;27:119–127.

41 Martos-Moreno GA, Barrios V, Argente J: Normative data for adiponectin, resistin, interleukin 6, and leptin/receptor ratio in a healthy Spanish pediatric population: relationship with sex steroids. Eur J Endocrinol 2006;155:429–434.

42 Suter KJ, Pohl CR, Wilson ME: Circulating concentrations of nocturnal leptin, growth hormone, and insulin-like growth factor-I increase before the onset of puberty in agonadal male monkeys: potential signals for the initiation of puberty. J Clin Endocrinol Metab 2000;85:808–814.

43 Bluher S, Mantzoros CS: Leptin in humans: lessons from translational research. Am J Clin Nutr 2009;89: 991S–997S.

44 Brandao CM, Lombardi MT, Nishida SK, Hauache OM, Vieira JG: Serum leptin concentration during puberty in healthy nonobese adolescents. Braz J Med Biol Res 2003;36:1293–6.

45 Clayton PE, Gill MS, Hall CM, Tillmann V, Whatmore AJ, Price DA: Serum leptin through childhood and adolescence. Clin Endocrinol (Oxf) 1997;46: 727–33.

46 Federico G, Baroncelli GI, Vanacore T, Fiore L, Saggese G: Pubertal changes in biochemical markers of growth. Horm Res 2003;60:46–51.

47 Matkovic V, Ilich JZ, Badenhop NE, et al: Gain in body fat is inversely related to the nocturnal rise in serum leptin level in young females. J Clin Endocrinol Metab 1997;82:1368–1372.

48 Maeda K, Okubo K, Shimomura I, Funahashi T, Matsuzawa Y, Matsubara K: cDNA cloning and expression of a novel adipose specific collagen-like factor, apM1 (AdiPose Most abundant Gene transcript 1). Biochem Biophys Res Commun 1996;221: 286–289.

49 Jeffery AN, Murphy MJ, Metcalf BS, et al: Adiponectin in childhood. Int J Pediatr Obes 2008;3:130–140.

50 Tsou PL, Jiang YD, Chang CC, et al: Sex-related differences between adiponectin and insulin resistance in schoolchildren. Diabetes Care 2004;27:308–313.

51 Martin TJ, Romas E, Gillespie MT: Interleukins in the control of osteoclast differentiation. Crit Rev Eukaryot Gene Expr 1998;8:107–123.

52 Bertolini DR, Nedwin GE, Bringman TS, Smith DD, Mundy GR: Stimulation of bone resorption and inhibition of bone formation in vitro by human tumour necrosis factors. Nature 1986;319:516–518.

53 Gaspersic R, Stiblar-Martincic D, Osredkar J, Skaleric U: Influence of subcutaneous administration of recombinant TNF-alpha on ligature-induced periodontitis in rats. J Periodontal Res 2003;38:198–203.

54 Aris RM, Stephens AR, Ontjes DA, et al: Adverse alterations in bone metabolism are associated with lung infection in adults with cystic fibrosis. Am J Respir Crit Care Med 2000;162:1674–1678.
55 Wennberg P, Nordstrom P, Lorentzon R, Lerner UH, Lorentzon M: TNF-alpha gene polymorphism and plasma TNF-alpha levels are related to lumbar spine bone area in healthy female Caucasian adolescents. Eur J Endocrinol 2002;146:629–634.
56 Rees A, Thomas N, Brophy S, Knox G, Williams R: Cross sectional study of childhood obesity and prevalence of risk factors for cardiovascular disease and diabetes in children aged 11–13. BMC Public Health 2009;9:86.
57 McTernan CL, McTernan PG, Harte AL, Levick PL, Barnett AH, Kumar S: Resistin, central obesity, and type 2 diabetes. Lancet 2002;359:46–47.
58 Li M, Fisette A, Zhao XY, Deng JY, Mi J, Cianflone K: Serum resistin correlates with central obesity but weakly with insulin resistance in Chinese children and adolescents. Int J Obes (Lond) 2009;33:424–439.
59 Gerber M, Boettner A, Seidel B, et al: Serum resistin levels of obese and lean children and adolescents: biochemical analysis and clinical relevance. J Clin Endocrinol Metab 2005;90:4503–4509.
60 Oh KW, Lee WY, Rhee EJ, et al: The relationship between serum resistin, leptin, adiponectin, ghrelin levels and bone mineral density in middle-aged men. Clin Endocrinol (Oxf) 2005;63:131–138.
61 Luk T, Malam Z, Marshall JC: Pre-B cell colony-enhancing factor (PBEF)/visfatin: a novel mediator of innate immunity. J Leukoc Biol 2008;83:804–816.
62 Araki S, Dobashi K, Kubo K, et al: Plasma visfatin concentration as a surrogate marker for visceral fat accumulation in obese children. Obesity (Silver Spring) 2008;16:384–388.
63 Jin H, Jiang B, Tang J, et al: Serum visfatin concentrations in obese adolescents and its correlation with age and high-density lipoprotein cholesterol. Diabetes Res Clin Pract 2008;79:412–418.
64 Haider DG, Holzer G, Schaller G, et al: The adipokine visfatin is markedly elevated in obese children. J Pediatr Gastroenterol Nutr 2006;43: 548–549.
65 Peng XD, Xie H, Zhao Q, Wu XP, Sun ZQ, Liao EY: Relationships between serum adiponectin, leptin, resistin, visfatin levels and bone mineral density, and bone biochemical markers in Chinese men. Clin Chim Acta 2008;387:31–35.
66 Blum WF: Leptin: the voice of the adipose tissue. Horm Res 1997;48(suppl 4):2–8.
67 Kettaneh A, Heude B, Oppert JM, et al: Serum adiponectin is related to plasma high-density lipoprotein cholesterol but not to plasma insulin-concentration in healthy children: the FLVS II study. Metabolism 2006;55:1171–1176.

Krista Casazza, PhD, RD
Department of Nutrition Sciences, University of Alabama at Birmingham
1530 3rd Ave S WEBB 415
Birmingham, AL 35294–3360 (USA)
Tel. +1 205 975 6226, Fax +1 205 934 7050, E-Mail kristac@uab.edu

Jürimäe J, Hills AP, Jürimäe T (eds): Cytokines, Growth Mediators and Physical Activity in Children during Puberty.
Med Sport Sci. Basel, Karger, 2010, vol 55, pp 32–42

Body Composition Differences in Normal Weight, Obese-Overweight and Anorexic Adolescents: Role of Adipocytokines

Kristin S. Ondrak · Anthony C. Hackney

Department of Exercise and Sport Science, Applied Physiology Laboratory, Fetzer Hall, University of North Carolina, Chapel Hill, N.C., USA

Abstract

Adipocytokines are signaling molecules released by adipose tissue with numerous functions, including regulation of metabolism, inflammatory process, and body mass. They are particularly interesting in youth, considering the rising prevalence of overweight/obesity and the linkage of this condition to inflammation. This chapter examines the relationship between body composition and select adipocytokines: leptin, adiponectin, IL-6, TNF-α, and resistin, in overweight, normal weight and anorexic youth. Leptin, which stimulates energy expenditure and promotes satiety, is highest in overweight youth, followed by normal weight and lastly anorexic youth. Adiponectin has similar functions to leptin but is negatively correlated with measures of body composition. Anorexic youth have the highest adiponectin per kg fat mass, followed by normal weight and overweight. Conversely, IL-6 is positively associated with body composition; however, research in anorexic youth is inconclusive. It has some pro-inflammatory effects and promotes glucose and fat use, therefore beneficial for maintenance of normal weight status. TNF-α is also a pro-inflammatory adipocytokine thought to be somewhat protective against cancer. TNF-α is highest in overweight, followed by normal weight and anorexic youth, similar to leptin. Finally, resistin is also involved in the pro-inflammatory response and the development of insulin resistance. However, far less research exists on this adipocytokine and its relation to body composition in overweight or anorexic youth is equivocal. In conclusion, several consistent relationships exist regarding adipocytokines and body composition; however, there is a need for additional research on these relationships in youth especially at extremes of adiposity such as overweight and anorexics.

Introduction

Adipocytokines are a collection of polypeptide signaling agents released from adipose tissue. Among their various functions, they are involved in energy balance (EB) and promote energy expenditure, appetite and satiety signals, as well as promote

Table 1. Typical adipocytokine levels in normal weight, overweight and anorexic youth

Adipocytokine	Normal weight	Overweight/obese	Anorexic
Leptin	3–16 ng/ml [7, 15–18, 20]	25–37 ng/ml [15–17]	2.5–4.6 ng/ml [15, 18–20]
Adiponectin	6.7–23.3 ng/ml [16–18, 20, 26–29]	5.8–18.6 ng/ml [16, 17, 26, 28, 29]	12.5–16.8 ng/ml [18, 20, 27]
IL-6	1.41–3.4 pg/ml [21, 28, 37]	1.78 pg/ml [28]	5.3 pg/ml [21]
TNF-α	1.35 pg/ml [28] to 3.85 pg/dl [29]	1.83–1.88 pg/ml [28] to 7.8 pg/dl [29]	no values located for anorexic youth
Resistin	3.5–10.1 ng/ml [7, 16, 28]	3.5–12.7 ng/ml [7, 16, 28]	no values located for anorexic youth

aspects of the inflammatory response. Adipocytokines also influence neuro-endocrine pathways within the body, such as the hypothalamic-pituitary-adrenal (HPA) axis and its subsequent effect on EB and overall metabolism [1]. They are also associated with many diseases such as osteoarthritis, rheumatoid arthritis, cardiovascular disease and obesity [2–6]. Relative to disease, adipocytokines have been linked to the development of insulin resistance and type 2 diabetes; in fact, leptin and interleukin-6 (IL-6) are positively correlated with glycolated hemoglobin (HbA_{1c}) levels in youth, which is a key marker of glucose control [7]. In addition to their potential roles to influence these diseases, adipocytokines are often influenced by factors such as biological age, pubertal stage, sex and may vary dramatically according to body composition. Considering the growing epidemics of obesity and related diseases in youth, it is especially important for researchers to understand how adipocytokines differ in accordance with body composition and weight status in youth. The purpose of this chapter is to examine this latter point and discuss how several common adipocytokines differ in youth with two extremes of body composition, those who are anorectic and overweight compared to those of a normal weight (NW) condition. The adipocytokines to be discussed in this chapter are limited to leptin, adiponectin, IL-6, tumor necrosis factor–alpha (TNF-α) and resistin. Table 1 depicts a summary of typical values found in the research literature of these selected adipocytokines of youth with varying body composition. Due to the extremely limited number of studies in children and adolescents on this topic, some related adult findings are discussed.

Anorexia nervosa (referred to as anorexia in this chapter) is a psychological disorder characterized by extreme loss of body weight due to food restriction and/or exercise. It is marked by severe energy deficits and a negative caloric balance that results in a body weight >15% below normal values for the individual's age and sex. Side effects of anorexia include decreased bone mineral density, electrolyte imbalances, and heart rhythm abnormalities. The majority of participants in research studies with anorexia are female, as the prevalence is higher than in males; for example, in the United States, 85–95% of those affected are female [8]. Researchers estimate that over the course of a female's life, 0.5–3.7% of the populace is likely to have anorexia [9]. Findings have shown that pro-inflammatory cytokines (e.g. TNF-α and IL-6) may play a key role in the development of the anorexia condition [1, 4, 10].

At the other extreme of body composition, being overweight is also associated with changes in several adipocytokines too. For the purposes of this chapter, overweight is defined as excessive body mass in relation to height; i.e. a body mass index (BMI) percentile ≥85th for the youth's age and sex. Becoming overweight results from positive EB, which may be attributable to excessive energy intake or low energy expenditure or both. Regrettably, the prevalence of overweight in youth has increased markedly in recent decades and current estimates show that 37.2% of 6- to 11-year-olds and 34.4% of adolescents aged 12–19 years have a BMI percentile >85th for their age and sex in the United States [11]. Furthermore, the World Health Organization (WHO) indicates the problem of overweight youth is not limited to the United States alone as many countries are experiencing an obesity epidemic [12]. The complications of being overweight are numerous and include predisposition to developing cardiovascular disease, orthopedic problems, type 2 diabetes, as well as altered blood lipid profiles and increased blood pressure.

Leptin

Discovered in 1994, leptin is a hormone released from adipose tissue. It has received a great deal of attention in the obesity literature due to its strong correlation with body weight and adipose tissue. Leptin has numerous target tissues throughout the body including the brain, where it increases energy expenditure and decreases hunger and related food intake [13]. Leptin acts as a critical link between adipose tissue and the reproductive system, indicating whether adequate energy reserves are present for normal reproductive function [14].

Leptin levels are higher in the overweight as the hormone is released by adipose tissue. It may appear counterintuitive that individuals who are overweight have increased levels of a hormone that promotes negative energy balance. However, overweight individuals commonly develop leptin resistance. Leptin also plays a role as a pro-inflammatory cytokine in the immune response. Furthermore, it is also associated with disease states such as insulin resistance and the subsequent development of type 2 diabetes, rheumatoid arthritis and osteoarthritis [13].

Research has shown increased leptin levels in overweight youth compared to their NW counterparts [7, 15–17]. Typical leptin values in NW youth ranged from 3 to

16 ng/ml [15–20], while overweight youth have substantially higher leptin levels of approximately 25–37 ng/ml [15–17]. In a study directly comparing pre-pubertal NW and obese youth, the latter had leptin values approximately five times greater (~25 vs. ~5 ng/ml, respectively) [15]. Similarly, Gerber et al. [16] compared lean and obese youth (mean BMI of 18.7 and 32.0, respectively) and found even larger group differences in leptin (3.0 vs. 34.3 ng/ml for lean and obese males; 6.5 vs. 36.7 ng/ml for lean and obese females, respectively). Other investigators reported a moderate strength correlation of 0.65 between leptin and body composition, quantified via BMI standard deviation scores, in this age population [15].

In contrast, youth with anorexia tend to have lower leptin values than NW youth, as would be expected [15, 18–21]. These relationships are also well established in young anorectic adults [22–25]. Typical leptin levels in youth with anorexia range from 2.5 to 4.6 ng/ml [15, 18–20]. The lower leptin values are consistent with the reduced body weight and body fat of individuals with anorexia, i.e. there is less adipose tissue to release leptin. Misra et al. [18] reported correlations of 0.66 between percent body fat and leptin in youth with anorexia; compared with 0.81 for NW youth. Other investigations have examined the effects of refeeding in patients with anorexia and found that leptin levels increased with gains in body weight [20, 26].

Therefore, this evidence supports that weight-related differences in leptin are seen in youth across the spectrum of body composition. Specifically, overweight youth tend to have the highest leptin values, followed by NW and lastly, anorexic.

Adiponectin

Adiponectin is an adipocytokine involved in EB and the promotion of energy expenditure, similar to leptin [6, 13]. Although, adiponectin is inversely related to the development of diseases such as rheumatoid arthritis, type 2 diabetes and cardiovascular disease and it is associated with reductions in some pro-inflammatory cytokines [13].

Adiponectin values tend to be somewhat higher in youth with NW compared to overweight or obese youth. For example, adiponectin values in youth with NW ranged from 6.7 to 23.3 ng/ml [16–18, 20, 27–30] while reported values for youth who were overweight were 5.8–18.6 ng/ml [16, 17, 27, 29, 30].

A significant correlation between adiponectin and percent body fat ($r = -0.44$) was found in a group of obese youth [31]. In this investigation, researchers examined the effect of weight loss in obese children on adiponectin levels and found increases (12.8–15.6 μg/ml) following significant weight loss (3.1 kg or 6% body fat in a 1 year period) [31]. Similarly, other authors have reported negative correlations between adiponectin and each of the following measures in NW youth: BMI percentile ($r = -0.48$), fat mass ($r = -0.43$), percent body fat ($r = -0.39$) [32], BMI ($r = -0.26$) [30] and visceral adipose tissue ($r = -0.53$) [27].

In contrast, adiponectin levels in girls with anorexia have been reported to range from 12.5 to 16.8 ng/ml [18, 20, 28], which are very similar to the values in girls with NW. However, when adiponectin levels are expressed per kilogram fat mass, girls with anorexia had *higher* levels compared to their NW counterparts [28]. In a study examining the effects of refeeding in individuals with anorexia, adiponectin levels declined following weight regain [20]. According to Qi et al. [6], this finding highlights the role of adiponectin as an indicator and protector of energy storage levels.

Several studies in adults have reported higher adiponectin levels in anorectic compared to NW individuals [22–25, 33, 34]. For example, Dolezalova [23] reported adiponectin values of 24.9 (±2.9) ng/ml in NW controls vs. 38.2 (±5.3) ng/ml in patients with anorexia. Interestingly, in this study, while circulating adiponectin was significantly elevated as a function of anorexia, subcutaneous fat adiponectin mRNA expression was decreased in the patients. The authors speculated this dissociation between subcutaneous expression and circulating adiponectin could be due to increased adiponectin production in other fat depots (i.e. visceral), or muscle tissue, or possibly an altered metabolic clearance rate in patients with anorexia.

Taken together, research on adiponectin in youth revealed that overweight youth have the lowest levels compared to NW. Anorexic are either similar to NW or have slightly greater levels than them when express relative to fat mass. However, when expressed per kg fat mass, adiponectin values are greater in anorexic youth as well as when comparing young anorexic adults to their NW counterparts.

Interleukin-6

IL-6 is a pro-inflammatory cytokine with numerous metabolic functions. These include the promotion of glucose uptake and synthesis of glycogen in skeletal muscle, as well as enhanced lipolysis and a related increased fat oxidation as an energy source [35]. These effects seem mediated by direct and indirect actions on the HPA axis [36]. Therefore, IL-6 is often thought to be 'protective' in a sense, against weight gain and the development of overweight status. In fact, research has shown when IL-6 was injected into mice, body mass and fat mass declined markedly [37].

In a study comparing NW, obese and diabetic Native American youth, IL-6 levels were highest in the diabetic group followed by those with obesity and NW (approximately 34, 26 and 19 pg/ml, respectively) [7]. Likewise, IL-6 was higher in youth with a larger waist circumference (>90th percentile), compared to those with a substantially smaller measurement (<75th percentile) [29]. However, IL-6 levels in the latter investigation did not differ between the two extremes of BMI nor sum of skinfolds (>95th vs. <75th percentile) in their populations. In a study of youth who were lean versus overweight, significant positive correlations were reported between IL-6 and BMI percentile ($r = 0.40$), percent body fat ($r = 0.46$) and fat mass ($r = 0.49$) [32].

In contrast to the above consistent findings, there have been mixed results regarding IL-6 levels in individuals with anorexia. For example, some researchers have reported that IL-6 is lower in youth with anorexia compared to NW youth [38], while others have reported higher values in girls with anorexia compared to those with NW [21]. It is unclear why these contradictions exist and are suggestive of the need for further research. Interestingly, in a refeeding study of participants with anorexia (aged 15–24 years), there was no change in IL-6 with body weight gain [26]. In adult subjects, researchers have also found mixed results with regard to IL-6 and anorexia. For example, Brambilla et al. [39] found no difference between these groups for IL-6 levels while others have reported trends for higher levels of IL-6 in adults with anorexia compared to NW participants [40, 41].

Viewed collectively, IL-6 tends to be higher in overweight youth compared to NW youth; however, the results with regard to anorexic youth (and adults) are mixed. Because of these equivocal results, it is not possible to draw firm conclusions at this time and additional research is needed on these relationships in anorexic youth.

Tumor Necrosis Factor-α

Tumor necrosis factor-α (TNF-α) is classified as a pro-inflammatory cytokine which has several key functions related to the immune response and development of inflammation [42]. As the name implies, TNF-α has been shown to lead to the necrosis (i.e. apoptotic cell death) of tumor cells and is therefore thought to be protective against some forms of cancer [42]. TNF-α is also able to act on the hypothalamus to produce fever, inhibit vascular smooth muscle tone (inducing low blood pressure), is a potent activator of endothelial coagulation, inhibits thrombomodulin, and inhibits tumorigenesis and some aspects of viral replication. Within skeletal muscle, it increases glucose use while decreasing liver glucose production thus leading to a lowering of blood glucose levels. It has also be referred to as 'cachexin' or 'cachectin' due to its association with the medical condition of 'cachexia', a wasting syndrome that causes muscular weakness and a loss of body weight, fat and muscle mass.

TNF-α levels are higher in youth who are overweight compared to NW youth [30, 43] and similar trends were found when body composition was delineated using either BMI or sum of skinfold (SSF) cutpoints (<75th vs. >95th percentile) [29]. Likewise, significant correlations have been reported between body composition, quantified in several ways, and TNF-α in youth; $r = 0.35$ (using BMI) [43], $r = 0.38$ (using BMI percentile) and $r = 0.45$ (using fat mass) [32]. Although, one investigation comparing youth with NW, obesity and diabetes reported similar TNF-α levels between groups, suggesting that TNF-α may *not* be related to body composition [7].

In youth with anorexia, however, TNF-α was found to be much lower when compared to a NW group [38]. In this study the participants with anorexia were treated (i.e. to increase body weight) in a hospital and upon release had even lower levels of TNF-α compared to their values at time of admission [38]. Other authors have also reported reductions in TNF-α following weight gain in participants with anorexia; however their results failed to reach statistical significance [26]. These findings are in stark contrast to a model presented by Holden and Pakula by which anorexia may result from elevations in TNF-α and changes in related neuropeptides, hormones and neurotransmitters [4]. To further complicate matters, relative to young adults, no differences were found when comparing TNF-α between individuals with anorexia and NW [39]. Taken together, these results suggest that the relationship of TNF-α to anorexia and overweight status is equivocal. Due to the relatively few studies in youth; however, it is difficult to draw informed conclusions at present.

Resistin

Resistin is another cytokine which plays a role in the body's inflammatory response and is associated with the development of insulin resistance [13]. Resistin is secreted by adipocytes (primarily the macrophage component) as well as mononuclear cells and epithelial cells. It is typically considered indicative of an overall state of inflammation in the body. The exact physiologic role of resistin is a subject of much controversy, however. Research suggests that resistin appears to cause tissues to be less sensitive to the action of insulin, which is a characteristic of type 2 diabetes. For this reason, there is a strong association in youth and adults between elevated levels of circulating resistin and type 2 diabetes and obesity.

In youth, resistin levels tend to be positively related to markers of body composition such as BMI, waist-to-hip ratio, waist circumference and percent body fat [5]. For example, resistin levels were higher in youth with a larger waist circumference (>90th percentile) compared to smaller waist circumference (<75th percentile) [29]. These latter findings point to resistin being related to the level of abdominal obesity as well as potentially to overweight status. This notion has been further supported by the Li et al. [5] who reported greater resistin levels in boys with central obesity. However, in a direct comparison of lean vs. obese children (mean age 12.5 years), resistin levels did not differ and ranged from ~5.7 to 6.8 ng/ml [16]. Stringer et al. [7] also reported no differences in resistin in youth with NW, obesity or diabetes, as all had levels of approximately 3.5 ng/ml. The resistin levels in the Li et al. [5] investigation just noted were higher, ~17.0 and 17.8 ng/ml for boys and girls with mean ages of 12.2 and 12.6 years, respectively [5]. Accordingly, there is considerable variability in absolute values of resistin in youth and inconsistencies in its relationship with body composition.

Unfortunately, we have been unable to locate any published research on the relationship between resistin and anorexia in children or adolescents. Therefore, we

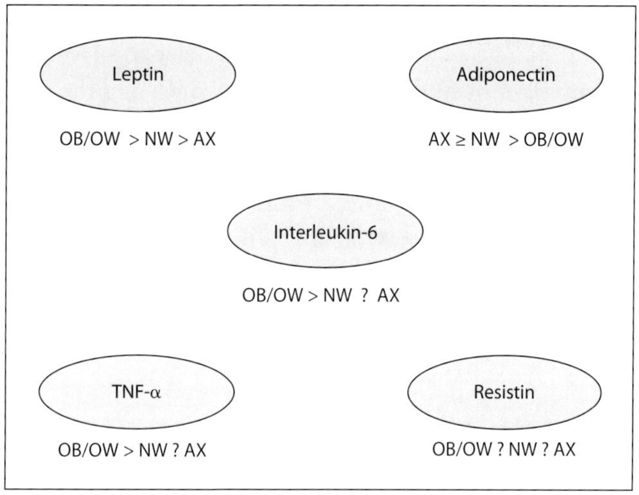

Fig. 1. Circulating levels of select adipocytokines vary across groups (obese-overweight, OB/OW, normal weight, NW, or anorexic, AX) of youth who are of different body compositions.

examined the adult literature on this topic where conflicting results were reported. For example, several studies reported no differences in resistin levels between NW and anorectic participants [23, 24, 33], while two reports showed that adults with anorexia had *lower* circulating resistin levels than NW adults [2, 34]. In contrast, researchers have also reported significantly higher levels of resistin measured in the extracellular space of adipose tissue in adults with anorexia compared to NW controls [2].

The lack of consistency in findings, and the limited number of studies, prevents us from drawing conclusions concerning weight-related differences in resistin in youth across the continuum of body composition. Therefore, further study is needed to investigate the relationship between resistin and anorexia, NW and overweight youth.

Conclusions

Research demonstrates that adipocytokines and body composition are related at the extremes of human adiposity (obesity vs. anorexia) in youth. Figure 1 is a schematic summary of these relationships as they are currently understood. The interactive nature of adipocytokines and adiposity is highly complex and has not been completely investigated. Thus, as indicated in the figure not all facets of the relationships have been fully delineated and are in need of further study.

Research clearly indicates that some adipocytokines are anorexigenic signaling agents that can lead to hypophagic behavior and subsequent negative EB, while other adipocytokines are orexigenic signally agents which can stimulate appetite and result in hyperphagia [10]. The reported change in some adipocytokine levels at the extremes of body composition may in fact stem from a particular eating behavior rather than be a causal factor in such behavior. However, due in large part to the limited number of studies in this area in youth and the constraints including ethical concerns when working with this population, it is impossible to be conclusive regarding the nature of the adipocytokine-body composition associations (i.e. causative, mediator, moderator). Substantially more research is needed to more completely characterize these associations and the potential cause-effect interaction within them. Such research will provide a clearer understanding of adipocytokines and their relation to adiposity in youth who vary in body composition status.

References

1 Corcos M, Guilbaud O, Paterniti S, Moussa M, Chambry J, Chaouat G, Consoli SM, Jeammet P: Involvement of cytokines in eating disorders: a critical review of the human literature. Psychoneuroendocrinology 2003;28:229–249.

2 Dostalova I, Kunesova M, Duskova J, Papezova H, Nedvidkova J: Adipose tissue resistin levels in patients with anorexia nervosa. Nutrition 2006;22: 977–983.

3 Gualilo O, Gonzalez-Juanatey JR, Lago F: The emerging role of adipokines as mediators of cardiovascular function: physiologic and clinical perspectives. Trends Cardiovas Med 2007;17:275–283.

4 Holden RJ, Pakula IS: The role of tumor necrosis factor-alpha in the pathogenesis of anorexia and bulimia nervosa, cancer cachexia and obesity. Med Hypotheses 1996;47:423–438.

5 Li M, Fisette A, Zhao X-Y, Deng J-Y, Mi J, Cianflone K: Serum resistin correlates with central obesity but weakly with insulin resistance in Chinese children and adolescents. Int J Obes (Lond) 2009;33:424–439.

6 Qi Y, Takahashi N, Hileman SM, Patel HR, Berg AH, Pajvani UB, Scherer PE, Ahima RS: Adiponectin acts in the brain to decrease body weight. Nat Med 2004;10:524–529.

7 Stringer DM, Sellers EA, Burr LL, Taylor CG: Altered plasma adipokines and markers of oxidative stress suggest increased risk of cardiovascular disease in First Nation youth with obesity or type 2 diabetes mellitus. Pediatr Diabetes 2009;10:269–277.

8 Andersen AE: Eating disorders in males; in Brownell KD, Fairburn CG (eds): Eating Disorders and Obesity: a Comprehensive Handbook. New York, Guilford Press, 1995, pp 177–187.

9 American Psychiatric Association Work Group on Eating Disorders: Practice guideline for the treatment of patients with eating disorders (revision). Am J Psychiatry 2000;157(1 suppl):1–39.

10 Wong S, Pinkney J: Role of cytokines in regulating feeding behavior. Current Drug Targets 2004;5:251–263.

11 Ogden CL, Yanovski SZ, Carroll MD, Flegal KM: The epidemiology of obesity. Gastroenterology 2007;32:2087–2102.

12 World Health Organization: Programmes and Projects: Global Strategy on Diet, Physical Activity and Health – Childhood Overweight and Obesity, 2009. http://www.who.int/dietphysicalactivity/childhood

13 Lago F, Dieguez C, Gómez-Reino J, Gualillo O: Adipokines as emerging mediators of immune response and inflammation. Nat Clin Pract Rheumatol 2007;3:716–724.

14 Moschos S, Chan JL, Mantzoros CS: Leptin and reproduction: a review. Fertil Steril 2002;77:433–444.

15 Argente J, Barrios V, Chowen JA, Sinha MK, Considine RV: Leptin plasma levels in healthy Spanish children and adolescents, children with obesity, and adolescents with anorexia nervosa and bulimia nervosa. J Pediatr 1997;131:833–838.

16 Gerber M, Boettner A, Seidel B, Lammert A, Bär J, Schuster E, Thiery J, Kiess W, Kratzsch J: Serum resistin levels of obese and lean children and adolescents: biochemical analysis and clinical relevance. J Clin Endocrinol Metab 2005;90:4503–4509.

17 Torres MD, Tormo MA, Campillo C, Carmona MI, Torres M, Reymundo M, García P, Campillo JE: Etiologic and cardiovascular risk factors in obese children from extremadura in Spain: their relationship with insulin resistance and plasma adipocytokine levels. Rev Esp Cardiol 2008;61:923–929.

18 Misra M, Miller KK, Almazan C, Ramaswamy K, Aggarwal A, Herzog DB, Neubauer G, Breu J, Klibanski A: Hormonal and body composition predictors of soluble leptin receptor, leptin, and free leptin index in adolescent girls with anorexia nervosa and controls and relation to insulin sensitivity. J Clin Endocrinol Metab 2004;89:3486–3495.

19 Misra M, Miller KK, Kuo K, Griffin K, Stewart V, Hunter E, Herzog DB, Klibanski A: Secretory dynamics of leptin in adolescent girls with anorexia nervosa and healthy adolescents. Am J Physiol Endocrinol Metab 2005;289:E373–381.

20 Modan-Moses D, Stein D, Pariente C, Yaroslavsky A, Ram A, Faigin M, Loewenthal R, Yissachar E, Hemi R, Kanety H: Modulation of adiponectin and leptin during refeeding of female anorexia nervosa patients. J Clin Endocrinol Metab 2007;92:1843–1847.

21 Misra M, Miller KK, Tsai P, Stewart V, End A, Freed N, Herzog DB, Goldstein M, Riggs S, Klibanski A: Uncoupling of cardiovascular risk markers in adolescent girls with anorexia nervosa. J Pediatr 2006; 149:763–769.

22 Delporte ML, Brichard SM, Hermans MP, Beguin C, Lambert M: Hyperadiponectinaemia in anorexia nervosa. Clin Endocrinol (Oxf) 2003;58:22–29.

23 Dolezalova R, Lacinova Z, Dolinkova M, Kleiblova P, Haluzikova D, Housa D, Papezova H, Haluzik M: Changes of endocrine function of adipose tissue in anorexia nervosa: comparison of circulating levels versus subcutaneous mRNA expression. Clin Endocrinol (Oxf) 2007;67:674–678.

24 Housova J, Anderlova K, Krizová J, Haluzikova D, Kremen J, Kumstyrová T, Papezová H, Haluzik M: Serum adiponectin and resistin concentrations in patients with restrictive and binge/purge form of anorexia nervosa and bulimia nervosa. J Clin Endocrinol Metab 2005;90:1366–1370.

25 Pannacciulli N, Vettor R, Milan G, Granzotto M, Catucci A, Federspil G, De Giacomo P, Giorgino R, De Pergola G: Anorexia nervosa is characterized by increased adiponectin plasma levels and reduced nonoxidative glucose metabolism. J Clin Endocrinol Metab 2003;88:1748–1752.

26 Vaisman N, Hahn T, Karov Y, Sigler E, Barak Y, Barak V: Changes in cytokine production and impaired hematopoiesis in patients with anorexia nervosa: the effect of refeeding. Cytokine 2004;26: 255–261.

27 Asayama K, Hayashibe H, Dobashi K, Uchida N, Nakane T, Kodera K, Shirahata A, Taniyama M: Decrease in serum adiponectin level due to obesity and visceral fat accumulation in children. Obes Res 2003;11:1072–1079.

28 Misra M, Miller KK, Cord J, Prabhakaran R, Herzog DB, Goldstein M, Katzman DK, Klibanski A: Relationships between serum adipokines, insulin levels, and bone density in girls with anorexia nervosa. J Clin Endocrinol Metab 2007;92:2046–2052.

29 Rubin DA, McMurray RG, Harrell JS, Hackney AC, Haqq AM: Do surrogate markers for adiposity relate to cytokines in adolescents? J Investig Med 2008;56: 786–792.

30 Shin JY, Kim SY, Jeung MJ, Eun SH, Woo CW, Yoon SY, Lee KH: Serum adiponectin, c-reactive protein and TNF-α levels in obese Korean children. J Pediatr Endoocrinol Metab 2008;21:23–29.

31 Reinehr T, Roth C, Menke T, Andler W: Adiponectin before and after weight loss in obese children. J Clin Endocrinol Metab 2004;89:3790–3794.

32 Nemet D, Wang P, Funahashi T, Matsuzawa Y, Tanaka S, Engelman L, Cooper DM: Adipocytokines, body composition, and fitness in children. Pediatr Res 2003;53:148–152.

33 Haluzíková D, Dostálová I, Kaválková P, Roubícek T, Mráz M, Papezová H, Haluzík M: Serum concentrations of adipocyte fatty acid binding protein in patients with anorexia nervosa. Physiol Res 2009;58: 577–581.

34 Krízová J, Dolinková M, Lacinová Z, Sulek S, Dolezalová R, Housová J, Krajícková J, Haluzíková D, Bosanská L, Papezová H, Haluzík M: Adiponectin and resistin gene polymorphisms in patients with anorexia nervosa and obesity and its influence on metabolic phenotype. Physiol Res 2008;57:539–546.

35 Hoene M, Weigert C: The role of interleukin-6 in insulin resistance, body fat distribution and energy balance. Obes Rev 2008;9:20–29.

36 Hackney AC, Battaglini CL, Evans ES: Cortisol, stress and adaptation during exercise training. Educ Phys Training Sport (Biomed Sci) 2008;3:34–41.

37 Jansson J, Wallenius K, Wernstedt I, Ohlsson C, Dickson SL, Wallenius V: On the site mechanism of action of the anti-obesity effects of interleukin-6. Grow Horm IGF Res 2003;13:S28-S32.

38 Nova E, Gómez-Martínez S, Morandé G, Marcos A: Cytokine production by blood mononuclear cells from in-patients with anorexia nervosa. Br J Nutr 2002;88:183–188.

39 Brambilla F, Monti D, Franceschi C: Plasma concentrations of interleukin-1-beta, interleukin-6 and tumor necrosis factor-alpha, and of their soluble receptors and receptor antagonist in anorexia nervosa. Psychiatry Res 2001;103:107–114.

40 Pomeroy C, Eckert E, Hu S, Eiken B, Mentink M, Crosby RD, Chao CC: Role of interleukin-6 and transforming growth factor-beta in anorexia nervosa. Biol Psychiatry 1994;36:836–839.

41 Raymond NC, Dysken M, Bettin K, Eckert ED, Crow SJ, Markus K, Pomeroy C: Cytokine production in patients with anorexia nervosa, bulimia nervosa, and obesity. Int J Eat Disord 2000;28:293–302.

42 Idriss HT, Naismith JH: TNF alpha and the TNF receptor superfamily: structure-function relationship(s). Microsc Res Tech 2000;50:184–195.

43 Moon YS, Kim DH, Song DK: Serum tumor necrosis factor-alpha levels and components of the metabolic syndrome in obese adolescents. Metabolism 2004;53:863–867.

Kristin S. Ondrak, PhD and Anthony C. Hackney, PhD
Department of Exercise and Sport Science, Applied Physiology Laboratory
CB# 8700, 209 Fetzer Hall, University of North Carolina
Chapel Hill, NC 27599 (USA)
Tel. +1 919 962 0017, Fax +1 919 962 0489, E-Mail kondrak@unc.edu

Jürimäe J, Hills AP, Jürimäe T (eds): Cytokines, Growth Mediators and Physical Activity in Children during Puberty.
Med Sport Sci. Basel, Karger, 2010, vol 55, pp 43–55

Inflammatory Cytokines and Metabolic Risk Factors during Growth and Maturation: Influence of Physical Activity

Daniela A. Rubin[a] · Anthony C. Hackney[b]

[a]Department of Kinesiology, California State University Fullerton, Fullerton, Calif., and [b]Department of Exercise and Sport Science, University of North Carolina, Chapel Hill, N.C., USA

Abstract

Cytokines influence tissue and cell physiology in positive and negative ways. Our aim in this chapter is to briefly present on select cytokines and their relationship to disease, metabolic risk factors, and physical activity in youth. We discuss the association of adiponectin, interleukin-6 (IL-6), resistin, tumor necrosis factor-α (TNF-α), and C-reactive protein (CRP) with metabolic risk factors in youth, and whether circulating concentrations of these cytokines are different based on being physically active or engaging in exercise training. Results from several studies show that adiponectin concentrations are reduced with increased adiposity, while others show that TNF-α, IL-6, resistin and CRP concentrations may be elevated with increased adiposity. Results from studies link decreased adiponectin with increased insulin resistance, while some evidence links increased TNF-α and resistin with increased insulin resistance. Several studies relate higher blood pressures to decreased adiponectin, increased TNF-α, and CRP concentrations. The only lipids associated with the cytokines appear to be triglycerides and HDL cholesterol. Higher levels of habitual physical activity are associated with higher adiponectin and perhaps decreased TNF-α and resistin concentrations. Exercise training also appears to positively influence the concentrations of these cytokines. In conclusion, the role of these cytokines is still somewhat unclear as is their associations with metabolic risk factors. However, the available evidence indicates that chronic inflammatory states such as obesity in childhood are associated with a pro-inflammatory profile and the presence of increased risk factors for disease while physical activity or exercise training elicit a protective role relative to this profile.

Introduction

This chapter presents an overview discussion on: (1) some key cytokines associated with cardiovascular disease and diabetes mellitus, (2) metabolic risk factors associated with cardiovascular and metabolic diseases, (3) the relationship between these cytokines and presented metabolic risk factors, (4) the relationship between physical activity and exercise training and inflammatory cytokines and metabolic risk factors, and (5) a possible link between physical activity, the select cytokines, and metabolic risk factors. The cytokines discussed include adiponectin, interleukin-6 (IL-6), resistin, tumor necrosis factor-α (TNF-α), and C-reactive protein (CRP). The metabolic factors that will be discussed are: indicators of overall adiposity, indicators of abdominal adiposity, concentrations of fasting plasma glucose and insulin, blood lipids, and blood pressure.

Key Inflammatory Cytokines and Their Role in Disease

The inflammatory cytokines form a complicated cascade of interacting mediators and modifiers of the inflammatory response to acute-chronic trauma and disease in humans. What follows is a brief introduction of some of the physiologic linkages and outcomes associated within the cytokines focused upon in this chapter.

Adiponectin is a protein (244 amino acid long polypeptide) that modulates a multitude of metabolic processes, including glucose regulation (increased muscle utilization) and fatty acid catabolism [1]. Adiponectin is exclusively secreted from the adipocyte of adipose tissue into the bloodstream. Because of its inverse relationship with adiposity and insulin resistance, low levels of it are associated with several major health problems such as type 2 diabetes mellitus (T2DM), obesity, atherosclerosis, nonalcoholic fatty liver disease and the 'metabolic syndrome' (see below).

Resistin is a protein (108 amino acid long, cysteine-rich polypeptide) secreted by adipocytes (primarily the macrophages component) as well as mononuclear cells and epithelial cells and is indicative of an overall state of inflammation. The physiologic role of resistin has been the subject of much controversy. Resistin does seem to cause tissues, especially the liver, to be less sensitive to the action of insulin [2], which is a characteristic of T2DM. Thus, there is a strong association in adults and youth between elevated levels of resistin with T2DM and obesity (i.e. most people with T2DM tend to be overweight or obese).

TNF-α (also called cachexin or cachectin) is a cytokine involved in systemic inflammation and is a member of a group of cytokines that stimulate the acute-phase reaction response and is considered highly pro-inflammatory. It is produced in monocytes, macrophages, T cells, myocytes and adipocytes. The primary role of TNF-α is in the regulation of immune cells, such as: stimulate recruitment of neutrophils and monocytes to sites of infection. Dysregulation and, in particular, overproduction of TNF-α have been implicated in a variety of human diseases such as hypertension, dyslipidemia, hyperinsulinemia, atherosclerosis, as well as cancer [3].

IL-6 is a cytokine that acts both as a pro-inflammatory and anti-inflammatory agent, a fact that has led to some confusion in the literature concerning interpretation of findings. It is secreted by T cells and macrophages (which can be within adipose tissue) to stimulate immune response to trauma or other tissue damage scenarios leading to an inflammation. However, IL-6 is also a 'myokine', a cytokine produced from muscle, and is elevated in response to skeletal muscle contraction and can thus serve as a signaling agent relative to metabolism. With exercise, it is substantially elevated and precedes the appearance of other cytokines in the blood [4]. During exercise, it is thought to act in a hormone-like manner to mobilize extracellular substrates and/or augment substrate delivery [5]. Smooth muscle cells in the tunica media of many blood vessels are also producers of IL-6, but its actions seem more pro-inflammatory with respect to this tissue. The role of IL-6 as an anti-inflammatory cytokine is mediated through its inhibitory effects on TNF-α and IL-1, and activation of IL-1ra and IL-10. IL-6 also seems to have some anabolic properties as it can induce the expression of endothelial growth factor. Elevations of IL-6 in the circulation stimulate CRP production in the liver, which has negative health outcomes (see below). Chronic circulating elevations IL-6 are associated with insulin resistance and a multitude of co-related health problems. However, some researchers consider IL-6 as a marker of metabolic dysregulation rather than a causative factor [6].

CRP is a protein found in the blood, the levels of which rise dramatically in response to inflammation and is considered part of an acute-phase reaction response. CRP is synthesized by the liver and its incremental increase is attributed to a rise in the plasma concentration of IL-6 and other signally factors released by adipocytes [7]. It is thought to assist in complement binding to foreign and damaged cells and enhances phagocytosis by macrophages, which express a receptor for CRP. When production is stimulated, its levels rise above normal limits within ~6 h, and typically peaks at 48 h. Exercise also results in an elevation of CRP in the circulation. Chronic elevations of CRP are associated with an increased risk of T2DM, hypertension, atherosclerosis and cardiovascular disease (CVD) [8].

Key Metabolic Risk Factors and Their Association with Disease

Obesity, abnormal glucose metabolism, altered lipid profile (elevated low-density lipoprotein [LDL] and triglycerides, and decreased high-density lipoprotein [HDL] cholesterol), and increased blood pressure have long been identified as precursors of either T2DM or CVD and adult mortality [9–11]. Of particular interest because of its increased prevalence, obesity is a key risk factor associated with increased impaired fasting glucose [12], increased blood pressure, and a dysregulated lipid profile [13, 14]. Studies have demonstrated that these risk factors cluster and, when clustering, the risk and severity of the disease increases [12, 15]. For example, adolescents who had impaired fasting glucose (fasting glucose ≥100–125 mg/dl) presented higher fasting insulin, total cholesterol, LDL, triglycerides, and systolic blood pressure (SBP), and lower HDL in comparison to those who had normal blood glucose concentrations [12].

This clustering of metabolic risk factors for T2DM and CVD has been defined as the metabolic syndrome [16, 17]. Because the presence of the metabolic syndrome in childhood predicts adult metabolic syndrome and diabetes 25–30 years later [17], the syndrome has been increasingly studied in youth. Studies evaluating the prevalence of the metabolic syndrome in United States and Europe have shown that the prevalence ranges from 0.2 to 9.4% depending on the cut-points used for criterion data [18, 19]. The most recent report evaluating data in the United Stated in adolescents showed that the prevalence of three risk factors was of 8.6% of the population, while 50% of them had at least one risk factor [18]. In European youth, the prevalence presented for metabolic syndrome was of 0.2 and 1.4% in children and adolescents, respectively [19]. About 15–20% of these youth had at least two risk factors or presented abdominal obesity [19]. Although the prevalence of the metabolic syndrome is difficult to determine, it appears that a large proportion of the pediatric population presents with at least one metabolic risk factor associated with preventable diseases.

Relationship between Metabolic Risk Factors and Cytokines

Obesity Surrogates (Increased Adiposity)

Several studies in youth have reported an association between higher adiposity levels, lower concentrations of adiponectin, and higher concentrations of IL-6, resistin, TNF-α, and CRP. A large number of studies have shown that even at young ages [20], children who are obese present lower adiponectin compared to their counterparts [21–23]. Differences in adiponectin are seen when youth are compared using BMI percentiles, percentage of ideal body weight [21], or waist circumferences percentiles [22]. Visceral adiposity appears to be more closely associated with adiponectin than overall adiposity [20]; that is, partial correlations between visceral adipose tissue and adiponectin are still significant ($r = -0.49$) even after adjusting for percentage of body fat. A few studies have shown either differences in IL-6 with increasing degree of obesity [23], or an association between IL-6 and surrogates of adiposity such as waist circumference [22]. However, weight reduction programs in youth have demonstrated that decreases in body mass also resulted in lower IL-6 concentrations in overweight children [24]. Because IL-6 is so highly variable, relatively large sample sizes are required to demonstrate differences related to obesity in this cytokine [23].

Only a few studies have demonstrated a large difference in TNF-α concentrations based on obesity. Moon et al. [25] showed a 3-fold difference in the concentrations of TNF-α between obese and nonobese adolescents. However, these authors indicated that the association between TNF-α and waist circumference was stronger than with BMI. Supporting these results, Rubin et al. [22] showed that in adolescents, those who presented abdominal obesity had ~20% higher TNF-α than those who did not; however, these authors failed to show differences based on BMI percentile. Other authors have recommended the use of TNF-α soluble receptors as markers of TNF-α because of their increased biostability. Consequently, two studies demonstrated higher concentrations of TNF-α receptors in overweight versus normal-weight children and adolescents [25, 26].

Only a limited number of studies have studied resistin concentrations in youth. Gerber et al. [27] failed to show significant differences based on BMI, and as did Rubin et al. [22]. This may be because of closer association between resistin and abdominal adipose tissue [28]. For example, Rubin et al. [22] presented ~25% higher resistin concentrations in those adolescents with a waist circumference higher than the 90th percentile compared to adolescents with a waist circumference lower than the 75th percentile. And similarly, Gerber et al. [27] demonstrated a significant positive association ($r = 0.21$) between waist circumference and resistin.

In a relatively small sample of adolescents and young adults ($n = 62$) Vikram et al. [29] showed that CRP was associated with BMI, and waist circumference. In a much larger study sample of girls and boys ($n = 3,846$), CRP was moderately associated with BMI percentile in girls ($r = 0.39$), and in boys ($r = 0.41$) [8]. Similarly, Weiss et al. [23] reported higher CRP concentrations in 439 severely obese participants compared to 30 nonobese siblings who served as the control sample. Increases in adiposity stimulate the production of IL-6 and TNF-α, and these cytokines in turn stimulate the production by the hepatocytes of CRP [30]. Thus, the association between BMI and CRP is not surprising.

Overall, many studies demonstrated either associations between BMI, BMI percentiles, percentage of body fat and these cytokines, or differences between overweight or obese and normal-weight youth. However, it appears that abdominal adiposity is more closely related with some of these cytokines than other indicators of relative adiposity such as BMI.

Fasting Glucose and Insulin (Indicators for Insulin Resistance)

As noted, adiponectin has been shown to affect glucose utilization and oxidation contributing to a decreased insulin resistance in the skeletal muscle and adipose tissue [1]. Therefore, it is not surprising that several cross-sectional studies demonstrated a negative relationship between fasting insulin (a surrogate for insulin resistance) and adiponectin [20, 21, 26, 31]. This association was demonstrated in cohorts of children with different degrees of body fat even when controlling for body fat, visceral adiposity, age and sex [21] as well as when analyses controlled for puberty or Tanner stage [26, 32]. Rubin et al. [31] also demonstrated that in their group of adolescents going through mid-puberty this association was stronger in overweight compared to normal-weight youth. In comparison to adiponectin, which is exclusively produced by adipose tissue, resistin is also produced by circulating monocytes. In a group of obese youth resistin was related weakly but significantly correlated (r = 0.18) with maximal insulin concentrations during an oral glucose tolerance test [27]. Interestingly, resistin concentrations in this last study were associated with testosterone, DHEAS, and estradiol as well as levels of Tanner stage [27]. Rubin et al. [31] demonstrated a positive relationship between insulin and resistin only in the boys of their study but not the girls. Although these investigators controlled for puberty (including youth in pubertal stages 2–4), they did not report controlling for steroid hormones [31].

Few studies have evaluated the associations between glucose or insulin and TNF-α or IL-6. Rubin et al. [31] reported a weak positive association between circulating TNF-α and fasting insulin, but no association with IL-6. However, the association with TNF-α disappeared when controlling for body fat as a possible confounder [31]. Lastly, Ford et al. [8] reported no significant association between fasting glucose and CRP.

Blood Lipids

Adiponectin stimulates utilization of fatty acids and their oxidation, and consequently production of triglycerides by the liver. If the circulating concentration of adiponectin is lower, such as in overweight or obese youth, the decreased levels of adiponectin may affect blood lipids status by the effect of a decreased fat oxidation rate. Therefore, it is of no surprise that studies in youth have shown that adiponectin is negatively associated with triglycerides in obese children [21], even in 2- to 6-year-olds [33]. However, as explained previously, this association seems mediated primarily by adiposity level [20]. In contrast, adiponectin appears positively associated with HDL [20] even when controlling for body fat, age, pubertal status and sex [32]. These results suggest that the latter association is not entirely dependent on levels of adiposity.

Mechanistic studies relate TNF-α with increased triglyceride production in the adipocyte by decreasing the activity of lipoprotein lipase and therefore stimulating lipogenesis. In obese adolescents, increased TNF-α concentrations are moderately associated with increased triglycerides [25]. In contrast, TNF-α is negatively correlated with HDL [25; Rubin et al., unpubl. obs.]. However, it appears that these associations are mediated by levels of body fat and its regional distribution as the associations are attenuated when controlling for waist circumference or BMI [Rubin et al., unpubl. obs.].

Unpublished research for our laboratory showed no associations between IL-6, or resistin and lipids [Rubin et al., unpubl. obs.]. Similarly, no significant associations have been shown between CRP and total cholesterol or triglycerides lipids [8] or between LDL and any of the cytokines of interest discussed here. Therefore, it appears that some but not all of these cytokines are related to lipid metabolism, and the parameters that show the strongest associations are triglycerides and HDL. However, future studies are needed to evaluate these associations.

Blood Pressure (Resting SBP and Ambulatory SBP)

Adiponectin (in vitro) modulates adhesion molecules gene expression in endothelial cells, reducing monocyte adhesion to the cells and preventing the development of lesions in the endothelium, which could be associated with atherosclerosis [34]. It could also modulate smooth muscle proliferation preventing increases in the intima media thickness [35]. Because of these anti-atherogenic properties for adiponectin, several studies in youth have investigated the relationship between adiponectin and blood pressure. A negative association between SBP and adiponectin was found in children, however, when the authors controlled for the effect of body fat using BMI as a surrogate, the association disappeared [26]. A similar finding was also reported by Bacha et al. [20]. However, in 68 adolescent females the association between SBP and adiponectin was significant even when controlling for other anthropometric variables [36]. Furthermore, in this study adolescents in the 3rd and 4th quartiles for SBP had significantly (~20%) lower adiponectin concentrations than those adolescents in the 1st SBP quartile [36].

Mechanistic studies suggest that TNF-α suppresses the release of nitric oxide (vasodilator) and therefore promotes increased vascular resistance and blood pressure [30]. However, in youth it appears that TNF-α is positively associated with SBP because of the association between body fat and SBP. This latter association was present only in obese but not in normal-weight or overweight adolescents [25].

Our unpublished data (referred to earlier) shows weak positive, yet significant, associations between both resistin and IL-6 and SBP ($r = 0.21$ and $r = 0.24$, respectively). Both associations are dependent on adiposity either expressed as BMI or waist circumference. In contrast, Gilardini et al. [37] failed to demonstrate an association between ambulatory SBP and IL-6 in obese children.

It has been shown that CRP affects the arteries of healthy children by disturbing endothelial function and stimulating intima media thickness (see earlier discussion). With increased intima media thickness the pressure inside the vessel increases, predisposing to tissue damage and build up of fibrous plaque [38]. However, the results of Ford [8] present a fairly weak association ($r = 0.20$) between SBP and CRP, both in girls and in boys. In a much smaller sample of overweight youth, those youth who presented hypertension ($n = 50$) had higher CRP concentrations in comparison to youth with similar percentage of body fat but without hypertension [39]. This study demonstrated the independent contribution of CRP, among other variables to the prediction of SBP in hypertensive youth only [39]. Therefore, the data shows a clear association between CRP concentrations and increased SBP in youth.

In comparison to adiponectin and CRP, there is still no conclusive data showing an association between TNF-α, resistin, and IL-6 and SBP in normal-weight youth. However, based on the information presented it also appears that in adolescents these associations are more evident. This would be expected as there is a longer time-course for interactions at the tissue level causing vessel stiffness and increases in blood pressure.

Association between Physical Activity/Exercise Training and Cytokines

The terms 'physical activity' and 'exercise training' are sometimes used interchangeably in the research literature. However, this is not always appropriate as they are not mutually inclusive. Exercise is more appropriately used to describe intentional muscular activity that is used as a means of elevating energy expenditure for the purposes of improving health and physical fitness level. Physical activity could encompass such activities, but is more typically representative of spontaneous or intentional muscular activity undertaken in carrying out recreational, work-related or events of daily living. It is also important to recognize that physical activity and exercise can be of an acute or chronic nature. Acute refers to a single session of physical activity and/or exercise and the consequent short-term effects and outcomes in response to that single session. In contrast, chronic refers to regular or frequent physical activity and exercise (i.e., training) undertaken over a prolonged period (over several weeks, months or years). For our purposes we will address both physical activity and exercise together, but will limit our discussion to chronic exposure effects.

Cross-sectional studies point to adiponectin levels being ~25–30% higher in adolescent girls who are physically active compared to sedentary or less active girls [40, 41]; although, not all such studies have shown this effect [42]. Balagopal et al. [43] showed in an intervention based study with obese adolescents a 34% increased in adiponectin levels with the introduction of 45 min of physical activity three times a week over a 3-month period. Similar results were shown in a later study [44].

Less research has dealt with resistin in youth. Nevertheless, Rubin et al. [41] have shown that adolescent boys who were of normal weight but with high levels of vigorous physical activity had substantially lower resistin levels than comparable boys who completed less vigorous physical activity. Some cross-sectional work supports the association between increased levels of physical activity in adolescents and decreased TNF-α levels [40], while similarly designed studies have shown little or no substantial effect on TNF-α or TNF-α soluble receptors [41, 42]. However, it is well demonstrated in adults that regular physical activity and exercise training typically results in lower TNF-α levels [6]. Several studies have demonstrated IL-6 to show a consistent reduction following exercise training [24, 25] or to be lower in children/youth who are more physically active [40, 42]. In these studies the magnitude of the effect of physical activity/exercise was such that IL-6 values were 26–49% lower. Finally, CRP has been shown to also be reduced (~30%) in intervention studies when physical activity or exercise training are introduced [43, 45]. However, the cross-sectional study by Platat et al. [42] found no effect of physical activity on CRP levels and a study by Kelly et al. [46] using 8 weeks of exercise

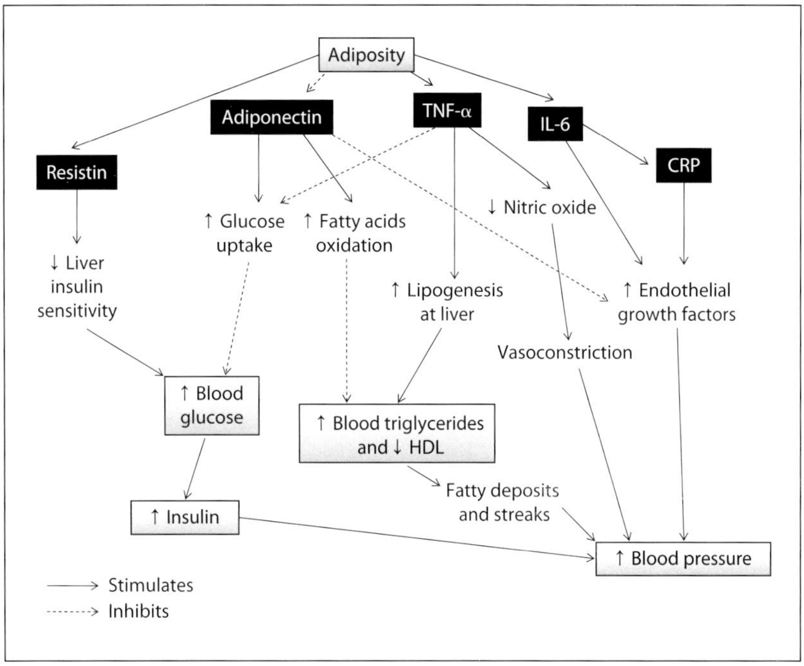

Fig. 1. Relationship between cytokines and metabolic risk factors. Key proposed mechanisms supporting these associations are presented.

training resulted in no change in CRP. The latter studies may, however, have been influenced by the fact that the activity-exercise levels completed were low in intensity and/or of short duration of training. Vigorous physical activity therefore seems to be a critical aspect in the performance of activity and exercise in order to impact upon some cytokines [41].

Associations between Physical Activity/Exercise Training and Metabolic Risk Factors

Although more research is needed to understand the association between physical activity and obesity in youth, the data are highly convincing regarding other metabolic risk factors. A meta-analysis of physical activity or exercise training studies in youth by Froberg and Andersen [47] showed that systolic and diastolic blood pressure, triglycerides, and insulin decreased with increased exercise while HDL increased. Similarly, another manuscript evaluating the dose of physical activity in youth required for such beneficial changes presented similar findings as well as recommendations for decreases [48] in adiposity [48]. In addition, a study using a large sample of European youth found a negative association between physical activity and development of the metabolic syndrome [19].

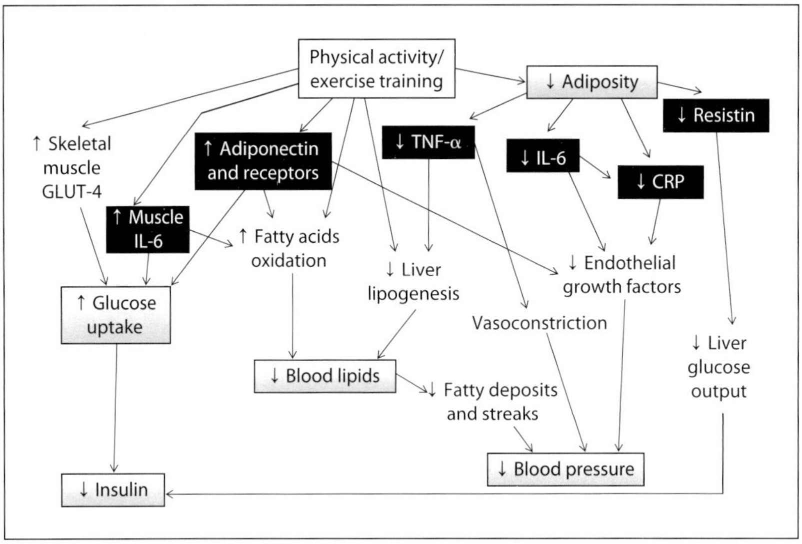

Fig. 2. Pathways and mechanisms mediating the influence of physical activity/exercise training on adiposity, cytokines and metabolic risk factors and their inter-relationships.

Final Hypothesis: Physical Activity Influences Adiposity, Cytokines, and Metabolic Risk Factors by Interdependent and Independent Mechanisms

As presented in previous sections, habitual physical activity, as well as exercise training positively influences some of the cytokines discussed. While one mechanism by which physical activity may increase adiponectin, and decrease the concentrations of TNF-α, IL-6, resistin and CRP is by reducing body fat mass; other studies in adults and youth support the existence of adiposity-independent mechanisms [40, 41]. That is, it is possible that habitual physical activity or exercise training influence the actions of these cytokines at the tissue level resulting in: (1) increased insulin sensitivity – particularly by increased adiponectin concentrations and decreased resistin concentrations, and decreased triglyceride output by the liver, and (2) lower blood pressure – because of cytokine-independent mechanisms related to decreased total peripheral resistance or cytokine-dependent mechanisms promoting vasodilation (e.g. increased adiponectin, and decreased TNF-α resulting on increased nitric oxide). Furthermore, studies in adults have proposed that exercise training lowers triglyceride concentrations by decreasing the output of very low density lipoprotein by the liver, and increasing the activity of lipoprotein lipase (LPL) in the adipose tissue [49]. Possibly, exercise also contributes to the increased LPL activity by suppressing the inhibiting action of TNF-α. The mechanisms linking exercise training and increased HDL have yet to be completely elicited [49]; but it is possible that cytokines have a role in this relationship since adiponectin is associated with increased HDL independent of changes in fat mass. Also, muscular contraction (i.e. acute physical activity exercise) causes the production and release of IL-6 from skeletal muscle [4]. The increase in IL-6 results in enhanced lipolysis and fat oxidation (directly via activation of AMPK; indirectly via its influence on cortisol) potentially impacting greatly on the lipid profile and the level of overall fat mass [4].

Obviously, the role of cytokines on inflammation, and metabolic risk in youth is an area where a continued line of research is needed as many questions remain unanswered. The increasing prevalence of childhood obesity and related comorbities throughout the world warrants further understanding of these relationships. More importantly is to acknowledge that the relationships discussed in this manuscript develop over a lifetime, and the metabolic actions of the cytokines should not be considered in isolation. Different cytokines could be acting and interacting at the same time on different tissues, resulting eventually in many disease-related consequences that could and should be prevented.

References

1 Yamauchi T, Kamon J, Minokoshi Y, et al: Adiponectin stimulates glucose utilization and fatty-acid oxidation by activating AMP-activated protein kinase. Nat Med 2002;8:1288–1295.

2 Steppan CM, Bailey ST, Bhat S, et al: The hormone resistin links obesity to diabetes. Nature 2001;409: 307–312.

3 Fernandez-Real JM, Ricart W: Insulin resistance and chronic cardiovascular inflammatory syndrome. Endocr Rev 2003;24:278–301.

4 Pedersen BK, Akerstrom TC, Nielsen AR, Fischer CP: Role of myokines in exercise and metabolism. J Appl Physiol 2007;103:1093–1098.

5 Pedersen BK, Febbraio MA: Interleukin-6 does have a beneficial role in insulin sensitivity and glucose homeostasis. J Appl Physiol 2007;102:814–826.

6 Petersen AM, Pedersen BK: The anti-inflammatory effect of exercise. J Appl Physiol 2005;98:1154–1162.

7 Pepys MB, Hirschfield GM: C-reactive protein: a critical update. J Clin Invest 2003;111:1805–1812.

8 Ford ES: C-reactive protein concentration and cardiovascular disease risk factors in children: findings from the National Health and Nutrition Examination Survey 1999–2000. Circulation 2003;108: 1053–1058.

9 Bjorge T, Engeland A, Tverdal A, Smith GD: Body mass index in adolescence in relation to cause-specific mortality: a follow-up of 230,000 Norwegian adolescents. Am J Epidemiol 2008;168:30–37.

10 Stokes J 3rd, Kannel WB, Wolf PA, D'Agostino RB, Cupples LA: Blood pressure as a risk factor for cardiovascular disease: the Framingham Study – 30 years of follow-up. Hypertension 1989;13:I13-I18.

11 Wilson PW, Abbott RD, Castelli WP: High density lipoprotein cholesterol and mortality: the Framingham Heart Study. Arteriosclerosis 1988;8: 737–741.

12 Williams DE, Cadwell BL, Cheng YJ, et al: Prevalence of impaired fasting glucose and its relationship with cardiovascular disease risk factors in US adolescents, 1999–2000. Pediatrics 2005;116:1122–1236.

13 Lee S, Bacha F, Gungor N, Arslanian SA: Waist circumference is an independent predictor of insulin resistance in black and white youths. J Pediatr 2006; 148:188–194.

14 Williams DP, Going SB, Lohman TG, et al: Body fatness and risk for elevated blood pressure, total cholesterol, and serum lipoprotein ratios in children and adolescents. Am J Public Health 1992;82:358–363.

15 McGill HC Jr, McMahan CA, Herderick EE, Malcom GT, Tracy RE, Strong JP: Origin of atherosclerosis in childhood and adolescence. Am J Clin Nutr 2000;72: 1307S–1315S.

16 Reaven GM: Banting lecture 1988. Role of insulin resistance in human disease. Diabetes 1988;37:1595–1607.

17 Morrison JA, Friedman LA, Wang P, Glueck CJ: Metabolic syndrome in childhood predicts adult metabolic syndrome and type 2 diabetes mellitus 25 to 30 years later. J Pediatr 2008;152:201–206.

18 Johnson WD, Kroon JJ, Greenway FL, Bouchard C, Ryan D, Katzmarzyk PT: Prevalence of risk factors for metabolic syndrome in adolescents: National Health and Nutrition Examination Survey (NHANES), 2001–2006. Arch Pediatr Adolesc Med 2009;163:371–377.

19 Ekelund U, Anderssen S, Andersen LB, et al: Prevalence and correlates of the metabolic syndrome in a population-based sample of European youth. Am J Clin Nutr 2009;89:90–96.

20 Bacha F, Saad R, Gungor N, Arslanian SA: Adiponectin in youth: relationship to visceral adiposity, insulin sensitivity, and beta-cell function. Diabetes Care 2004;27:547–552.

21 Asayama K, Hayashibe H, Dobashi K, et al: Decrease in serum adiponectin level due to obesity and visceral fat accumulation in children. Obes Res 2003; 11:1072–1079.

22 Rubin DA, McMurray RG, Harrell JS, Hackney AC, Haqq AM: Do surrogate markers for adiposity relate to cytokines in adolescents? J Invest Med 2008;56: 786–792.

23 Weiss R, Dziura J, Burgert TS, et al: Obesity and the metabolic syndrome in children and adolescents. N Engl J Med 2004;350:2362–2374.

24 Gallistl S, Sudi KM, Cvirn G, Muntean W, Borkenstein M: Effects of short-term energy restriction and physical training on haemostatic risk factors for coronary heart disease in obese children and adolescents. Int J Obes Relat Metab Disord 2001;25:529–532.

25 Moon YS, Kim DH, Song DK: Serum tumor necrosis factor-alpha levels and components of the metabolic syndrome in obese adolescents. Metabolism 2004;53:863–867.

26 Chu NF, Shen MH, Wu DM, Lai CJ: Relationship between plasma adiponectin levels and metabolic risk profiles in Taiwanese children. Obes Res 2005; 13:2014–2020.

27 Gerber M, Boettner A, Seidel B, et al: Serum resistin levels of obese and lean children and adolescents: biochemical analysis and clinical relevance. J Clin Endocrinol Metab 2005;90:4503–4509.

28 McTernan CL, McTernan PG, Harte AL, Levick PL, Barnett AH, Kumar S: Resistin, central obesity, and type 2 diabetes. Lancet 2002;359:46–57.

29 Vikram NK, Misra A, Pandey RM, Dwivedi M, Luthra K: Adiponectin, insulin resistance, and C-reactive protein in postpubertal Asian Indian adolescents. Metabolism 2004;53:1336–1341.

30 de Ferranti S, Mozaffarian D: The perfect storm: obesity, adipocyte dysfunction, and metabolic consequences. Clin Chem 2008;54:945–955.

31 Rubin DA, McMurray RG, Harrell JS, Hackney AC, Thorpe DE, Haqq AM: The association between insulin resistance and cytokines in adolescents: the role of weight status and exercise. Metabolism 2008; 57:683–690.

32 Huang KC, Lue BH, Yen RF, et al: Plasma adiponectin levels and metabolic factors in nondiabetic adolescents. Obes Res 2004;12:119–124.

33 Cianflone K, Lu H, Smith J, Yu W, Wang H: Adiponectin, acylation stimulating protein and complement C3 are altered in obesity in very young children. Clin Endocrinol (Oxf) 2005;62:567–572.

34 Ouchi N, Kihara S, Arita Y, et al: Novel modulator for endothelial adhesion molecules: adipocyte-derived plasma protein adiponectin. Circulation 1999;100:2473–2476.

35 Kubota N, Terauchi Y, Yamauchi T, et al: Disruption of adiponectin causes insulin resistance and neointimal formation. J Biol Chem 2002;277:25863–25866.

36 Huang KC, Chen CL, Chuang LM, Ho SR, Tai TY, Yang WS: Plasma adiponectin levels and blood pressures in nondiabetic adolescent females. J Clin Endocrinol Metab 2003;88:4130–4134.

37 Gilardini L, Parati G, Sartorio A, Mazzilli G, Pontiggia B, Invitti C: Sympathoadrenergic and metabolic factors are involved in ambulatory blood pressure rise in childhood obesity. J Hum Hypertens 2008;22:75–82.

38 Jarvisalo MJ, Harmoinen A, Hakanen M, et al: Elevated serum C-reactive protein levels and early arterial changes in healthy children. Arterioscler Thromb Vasc Biol 2002;22:1323–1328.

39 Garanty-Bogacka B, Syrenicz M, Syrenicz A, Gebala A, Lulka D, Walczak M: Serum markers of inflammation and endothelial activation in children with obesity-related hypertension. Neuro Endocrinol Lett 2005;26:242–246.

40 Ischander M, Zaldivar F Jr, Eliakim A, et al: Physical activity, growth, and inflammatory mediators in BMI-matched female adolescents. Med Sci Sports Exerc 2007;39:1131–1138.

41 Rubin DA, McMurray RG, Harrell JS, Thorpe DE, Hackney AC: Vigorous physical activity and cytokines in adolescents. Eur J Appl Physiol 2008;103:495–500.

42 Platat C, Wagner A, Klumpp T, Schweitzer B, Simon C: Relationships of physical activity with metabolic syndrome features and low-grade inflammation in adolescents. Diabetologia 2006;49:2078–2085.

43 Balagopal P, George D, Yarandi H, Funanage V, Bayne E: Reversal of obesity-related hypoadiponectinemia by lifestyle intervention: a controlled, randomized study in obese adolescents. J Clin Endocrinol Metab 2005;90:6192–6197.

44 Kim ES, Im JA, Kim KC, et al: Improved insulin sensitivity and adiponectin level after exercise training in obese Korean youth. Obesity (Silver Spring) 2007;15:3023–3030.
45 Rosenbaum M, Nonas C, Weil R, et al: School-based intervention acutely improves insulin sensitivity and decreases inflammatory markers and body fatness in junior high school students. J Clin Endocrinol Metab 2007;92:504–508.
46 Kelly AS, Steinberger J, Olson TP, Dengel DR: In the absence of weight loss, exercise training does not improve adipokines or oxidative stress in overweight children. Metabolism 2007;56:1005–1009.
47 Froberg K, Andersen LB: Mini review: physical activity and fitness and its relations to cardiovascular disease risk factors in children. Int J Obes 2005; 29(suppl 2):S34–S39.
48 Strong WB, Malina RM, Blimkie CJ, et al: Evidence based physical activity for school-age youth. J Pediatr 2005;146:732–737.
49 Chan DC, Barrett PH, Watts GF: Recent studies of lipoprotein kinetics in the metabolic syndrome and related disorders. Curr Opin Lipidol 2006;17:28–36.

Daniela A. Rubin, PhD
California State University Fullerton
800 N. State College Blvd.
Fullerton, CA, 92834 (USA)
Tel. +1 657 278 4704, Fax +1 657 278 5317, E-Mail drubin@fullerton.edu

Jürimäe J, Hills AP, Jürimäe T (eds): Cytokines, Growth Mediators and Physical Activity in Children during Puberty.
Med Sport Sci. Basel, Karger, 2010, vol 55, pp 56–68

Visfatin and Adiponectin Levels in Children: Relationships with Physical Activity and Metabolic Parameters

Jarek Mäestu · Jaak Jürimäe · Toivo Jürimäe

Faculty of Exercise and Sport Sciences, Centre of Behavioral and Health Sciences, University of Tartu, Tartu, Estonia

Abstract

Childhood obesity is increasing throughout the world and increases in adipose tissue are related to insulin resistance, cardiovascular diseases and metablic syndrome. Adipose tissue is not simply a storage depot for surplus energy but rather, is an active organ that modulates various biological functions and synthesizes and secretes multiple cytokines into the circulation. Adiponectin and visfatin are two cytokines which are considered to be possible links between obesity, insulin resistance and the metabolic syndrome. In turn, concentrations of adiponectin and visfatin are mainly influenced by the overall body fat mass which is one of the main determinants of insulin resistance and cardiovascular diseases. In contrast, physical activity and exercise are negatively related to body fat mass and also have an influence on cytokine concentrations in the blood. It is of particular interest whether physical activity or lifestyle interventions have a positive effect on adiponectin and visfatin concentrations in the blood. The aim of this review is to provide an overview of the contribution of vistafin and adiponectin to various metabolic parameters and their relationship with different physical activity patterns in children and adolescents.

The increasing prevalence of obesity is becoming an important public health problem in childhood and presents numerous problems during adolescence and adulthood. Obesity is of particular concern because it drives the insulin resistance that is believed to underlie diabetes, cardiovascular disease, and the metabolic syndrome [1]. However, the link between adipose tissue and the increased resistance to insulin is still unclear. During puberty, there is an increase in insulin resistance that may be related to changes in growth hormone, sex hormones, and increases in and redistribution of body fat [1]. Similar to the risks of obesity in adulthood, childhood obesity is a leading cause of pediatric hypertension associated with type II diabetes, and increases the risk of cardiovascular diseases [2]. Importantly, physical inactivity appears to be one of the main risk factors for cardiovascular disease [3].

The main roles of human adipose tissue are fuel storage, thermal insulation, and mechanical protection. However, adipose tissue is also now recognized as an endocrine organ which releases many cytokines such as leptin, tumor necrosis factor-α (TNF-α), interleukin-6 (IL-6), resistin, adiponectin and visfatin [2, 4]. The production, release and plasma concentrations of these adipose tissue-derived cytokines have been investigated extensively in healthy normal-weight [5, 6], obese [7, 8] and also physically active [3, 9] children and adolescents. Typically, the production of these molecules is increased with obesity, except adiponectin which is decreased [4]. Excess adiposity, the most common cause of insulin resistance in children [5, 10], may influence the association between these cytokines and insulin resistance [3, 8]. Undoubtedly, obesity, inflammation and cardiovascular disease seem to be closely linked, but it is difficult to establish the specific relationships between them. The simple assumption is that obesity-induced inflammation is a causal factor for cardiovascular diseases [11]. Among the cytokines, adiponectin and visfatin are thought to represent the link between adiposity and insulin resistance [9, 12].

Adiponectin, first identified in 1995, is one of the most abundant circulating adipose tissue-specific cytokines which is mainly produced by visceral adipose tissue [13] and is negatively regulated in obesity, diabetes and cardiovascular disease [14]. It circulates in high concentrations as a multimer, has a structural homology to TNF-α, and its receptors are highly expressed in liver and muscle [15]. Circulating adiponectin levels are tightly controlled and remain relatively constant [16]. Adiponectin has known direct and indirect functions [17] primarily related to endothelial function, the promotion of insulin sensitivity and inhibition of inflammatory mediators [17]. The primary factor found to be closely related to adiponectin concentration is the level of obesity. Adiponectin levels are decreased in obesity and are consistently reported as <6 μg/ml in obese individuals [18, 19]. This reduction in adiponectin appears to precede the disorders, and low levels of adiponectin have been shown to predict the development of type 2 diabetes and cardiovascular disease [20]. Lower amounts of adipose tissue, on the other hand, result in increased adiponectin expression with accompanying improvements in insulin sensitivity. Adiponectin also acts with insulin to inhibit hepatic glucose production whereas the globular domain stimulates fatty acid oxidation in skeletal muscle and other tissues [15]. It also decreases indirectly the levels of C-reactive protein (CRP) and IL-6 through the dose-dependent, reciprocal inhibition of TNF-α [21]. Adiponectin is also thought to improve insulin sensitivity and to have anti-inflammatory properties.

Visfatin, also known as pre-B cell colony-enhancing factor, is a cytokine that is also highly expressed in visceral adipose tissue [22]. The overall production of visfatin in the body can be attributed to bone marrow, liver, muscle, and peripheral blood mononuclear cells in addition to visceral adipose tissue [23]. Plasma levels of visfatin correlate with the amount of visceral fat in humans [7], in contrast to the rather weak relationship between visfatin and subcutaneous adipose tissue [24]. Growing evidence indicates a role for visfatin in glucose homeostasis [24]. It has also been suggested that the elevation of plasma visfatin concentrations in obese children may be independently involved in the development of metabolic syndrome and precede abnormal glucose tolerance [24]. Accordingly, increasing evidence supports the participation of this cytokine in inflammatory processes. Vistafin has been shown to stimulate IL-6 and IL-8; however, proinflammatory cytokines such as TNF-α and IL-6 have been shown to increase or downregulate visfatin synthesis [25, 26].

The aim of this review is to provide an overview of the contribution of adiponectin and visfatin to different metabolic parameters and their relationships with various physical activity patterns.

Adiponectin Concentrations in Childhood and Relationships with Metabolic Parameters

Adiponectin has been linked as a candidate mediator in the development of obesity-related insulin resistance during adolescence and adulthood. During puberty, girls in general have higher adiponectin concentrations than boys and concentrations decrease with age [27, 28]. Further, limited data suggest that adiponectin is 33% lower in obese children with diabetes than in those without diabetes [29]. Adiponectin has been reported to be negatively correlated with androgen concentrations, especially with testosterone in boys [27, 30]. Longitudinal studies in adults suggest that low adiponectin is a risk factor for type 2 diabetes: adiponectin concentrations are 22% lower in adults who subsequently develop diabetes than in those who do not [20]. However, Rubin et al. [31] showed that in overweight children an increase in adiponectin predicted an increase in insulin resistance at higher rate than in normal-weight subjects, suggesting that a protective role of adiponectin on insulin resistance is more relevant on overweight youths. The authors speculated that due to normal concentrations of triglycerides and other pro-inflammatory cytokines the protective role of adiponectin is minimal in contrast to obesity where adiponectin's protective role might be superseded by triglycerides and proinflammatory cytokines.

In general, adiponectin appears to be negatively related to insulin concentration [32] and insulin resistance [33], although Ong et al. [34] suggested a weak positive association for adiponectin in boys. In addition, the negative association between adiponectin and insulin resistance has been found to be independent of adiposity [35]. In contrast, no independent effect of adiponectin on markers of insulin resistance was found in a population-based sample of 1,632 9- to 16-year-old boys and girls [28]. In combination with the association between normal fat accrual and lower adiponectin during the pubertal years, the authors suggested that there may be mechanisms to reduce the effects of low adiponectin on insulin resistance [28]. These contrary findings might be explained by different populations with different values of fat mass, insulin sensitivity, and disease. The existence of a stronger association between adiponectin and insulin resistance with increasing adiposity could also partly explain these discrepancies [28]. Moreover, mouse models treated with adiponectin showed that adiponectin protects against insulin resistance to a greater degree in obese than normal-weight mice [36]. In children, adiponectin concentrations modified the relationship between BMI and fasting insulin score [28] and morbidly obese patients have demonstrated higher adiponectin values than obese patients [37]. However, this relationship in children should be further tested with more accurate measures of body fat mass. The involvement of TNF-α has also been shown to correlate with obesity in obese subjects, since TNF-α expression in adipocytes is suppressed by adiponectin [38]. Likewise, a study of human adipose tissue showed that subjects with the highest levels of adiponectin mRNA expression secrete the lowest levels of TNF-α [39]. Hotta et al. [40] showed a significant increase in adiponectin levels in both diabetic and non-diabetic patients after prolonged diet induced weight loss, with the diabetic subjects tending to have a greater absolute increase in adiponectin levels. Similar results were found by Monzillo et al. [41] who showed that after lifestyle intervention, adiponectin increased only in diabetic patients.

The relationships between adiponectin concentration and adipose tissue have been reported to be similar for measured overall and central adiposity indices in regularly physically active adolescents [9], whereas other studies have indicated that central fat distribution is a better determinant of circulating adiponectin than total fat mass in heterogeneous groups of adolescent children [42]. Furthermore, an independent association of plasma adiponectin concentration with fat-free mass (FFM) has been observed in physically active pubertal girls [9]. FFM, together with trunk fat and total fat mass values, have been found to characterize circulating adiponectin concentration by 84% ($R^2 \times 100$) in a multivariate analysis [9]. These findings suggest that in addition to body adipose tissue values, other body composition factors may modulate plasma adiponectin levels, at least in regularly physically active pubertal girls (table 1).

Visfatin Concentrations in Childhood and Relationships with Metabolic Parameters

Visfatin has been identified as a link between visceral obesity and type 2 diabetes mellitus [24, 43] due to visceral obesity being a risk factor for the development of insulin resistance and type 2 diabetes mellitus [22, 44]. However, some investigations have found no difference in the expression of visfatin in visceral and subcutaneous adipose tissue [45–47]. Furthermore, Varma et al. [47] revealed that visfatin is highly expressed in subcutaneous adipose tissue in relatively lean and more insulin sensitive individuals. Previous studies of visfatin in children and adolescents have also provided somewhat conflicting results. For example, a significant positive association between plasma visfatin and body mass index (BMI) has been suggested in some

Table 1. Factors that may modulate plasma adiponectin and visfatin concentrations in children

Cytokine	Possible factors influencing cytokine levels
Adiponectin	puberty↓ abdominal adipose tissue↓ overall adiposity↓ insulin↓ insulin resistance↓ weight loss↑ fat-free mass↑ physical activity↑ aerobic power↑
Visfatin	puberty? abdominal adipose tissue? overall adiposity↑ insulin↑ insulin resistance↑ weight loss↓ fat-free mass? physical activity? aerobic power?

studies [44], while others have reported no correlation between visfatin and indices of overall adiposity [5, 7, 24]. In addition, Fernandez-Real et al. [48] reported an independent association between visfatin concentration and insulin resistance in healthy lean adults, while previous studies in children have reported no independent relationship between visfatin and insulin resistance in physically inactive obese children and adolescents [5, 7, 24].

An independent association between visfatin concentration and insulin resistance has been reported in regularly physically active adolescent females [9], which contrasts with findings in inactive obese children and adolescents [7, 24]. Studies have also reported that in obese children visfatin concentrations in blood are related to anthropometric parameters, insulin, and insulin resistance, while no correlations were found in the nonobese group of children [7, 44]. However, similar relationships are not seen in population-based samples in adults [45, 46, 49–51]. Therefore, it has been suggested there is a threshold in childhood obesity above which relationships with adiponectin and indices of insulin resistance may have been more prominent [44].

Elevated levels of visfatin, similar to in the obese, have also been reported in patients with type 1 diabetes mellitus. Therefore, it has been suggested that visfatin does not play a specific role in the pathogenesis of the metabolic syndrome because type 1 diabetes mellitus originates from different pathophysiologies [52]. Plasma visfatin was also higher in lean type 1 diabetes mellitus patients compared to controls [52]. It was suggested that elevated plasma visfatin may be a consequence of intermittent or continued hyperglycemia or lack of physiological insulin exposure and may represent a feedback mechanism of glucose homeostasis [52].

It is not yet known by which mechanism visfatin is transported into the circulation since there is no signal sequence in their primary structure in order to be secreted into the circulation via endoplasmic reticulum mediated process in contrast to other peptide hormones [53].

It has been indicated that polymorphisms in the visfatin gene are associated with triglyceride and total cholesterol levels [54], which could suggest visfatin also has a role in lipid metabolism, which might be an important factor considering the effects of habitual physical activity and physical training on visfatin. Although higher blood lipid levels are usually found in obese children compared to nonobese children, correlations with visfatin have not commonly been found [24, 44]. Some studies, however, have found correlations between visfatin and HDL cholesterol [5, 24, 51]. These discrepant findings are difficult to explain however, different levels of adiposity and also the intensity and duration of physical activity levels of the subjects may be significant factors in visfatin concentration.

Adiponectin Responses to Acute Exercise and Chronic Physical Activity

It is widely recognized that lifestyle intervention with a modification of dietary habits and increased physical activity is the most important approach to address excess body fat in childhood and adolescence [41]. Exercise training influences vascular and metabolic cardiovascular risk factors including insulin resistance [55] and exerts effects on glycemic profile in subjects with type 1 or 2 diabetes. The mechanisms by which physical activity improves metabolic health are not completely understood. Given that metabolic disease is believed to be an inflammatory state there is considerable interest in the role of physical activity on metabolic health. Excess adiposity, the most common cause of insulin resistance in children, may influence the association between adipocytokines and insulin resistance [8]. However, since adipocytokines appear to respond to acute and chronic exercise [9, 32, 56], regular physical activity may also modify the association between adipocytokines and insulin resistance.

Adiponectin has been implicated in the regulation of energy homeostasis [36]. Platat et al. [57] in a study of 640 12-year-old adolescents, demonstrated that regular physical activity is inversely related to insulin levels and insulin resistance independent of adiposity and location of fat. However, they indicated that adipocytokines do not substantially contribute to the beneficial relationships of physical activity with insulin resistance. Exercise alone has been reported to increase circulating adiponectin levels significantly in adults [58–60]; however, studies have not generally controlled for caloric intake or dietary composition, potentially compromising the validity of attributing changes to adiponectin alone. Some authors have suggested that an increase in adiponectin concentration after exercise is prevalent if the energy expenditure is high enough [60]. However, the effect of training on circulating adipokines is inconsistent. For example, in adults, adiponectin concentrations have been found to increase [61], decrease [62], or remain unaltered [63] and prospective studies on training during puberty are clearly lacking in the literature. The impact of aerobic training on insulin and adiponectin on overweight and obese girls showed improved insulin sensitivity without changes in body weight, body fat, and adiponectin in a training program of 12 weeks and 3 days per week [64]. However, FFM increased, particularly in the lower extremity, and it was strongly associated with enhanced insulin sensitivity. As the skeletal muscle is the primary target tissue for insulin action, the authors suggested that the exercise training-induced increase in muscle mass may, at least in part, explain the enhanced insulin sensitivity [64]. However, we could suggest that the study population and training regimen for future training studies during puberty should be very precisely determined. Since adiponectin response to various types of training depends on different independent factors (i.e. body composition, muscle mass, diabetes, obese or athletes, sex of the subjects) these factors should be considered.

To date, adiponectin has received less attention with the respect to physical activity compared to the traditional metabolic markers in children. Although adiponectin has been found to be negatively related with insulin resistance, studies in adults have shown that there is no significant relationship between changes in insulin sensitivity and adiponectin concentrations [60, 65, 66]. In a cross-sectional study of 120 pubertal boys and girls, the higher levels of habitual vigorous physical activity and maximal aerobic power were correlated with increased adiponectin [31].

Cambuli et al. [67] studied 104 prepubertal and pubertal obese children and 54 controls in a 1-year lifestyle intervention and showed positive changes in clinical and metabolic parameters including adiponectin without weight loss with obese children. Adiponectin levels were similar to those of the normal-weight controls at the end of the study confirming the positive impact of the lifestyle intervention.

Metcalf et al. [12] showed that adiponectin was inversely related to physical activity even after adjustment for body fat and diet quality as adiponectin levels were higher in the least active tertile of nonobese prepubertal children. This is interesting because lower metabolic risk in children is associated with higher physical activity [68] and higher adiponectin level [9, 33]. Similarly, Yatagai et al. [62] showed that serum adiponectin decreased significantly in response to a 6-week exercise training program in men accompanied by decrease in insulin resistance without change in fasting insulin. The authors suggested that increased insulin action induced by exercise may suppress the expression and/or secretion of adiponectin. Metcalf et al. [12] further suggested that in conditions of low physical activity for the maintenance of insulin sensitivity, adiponectin may be secreted to compensate. In adults, it has also been found that exercise decreased insulin resistance without changing adiponectin [18].

Visfatin Responses to Acute Exercise and Chronic Physical Activity

Compared to adiponectin, the relationship of vistafin to physical activity has received far less attention in the literature. Furthermore, to the best of our knowledge, there are no longitudinal studies on exercise or lifestyle intervention and visfatin concentrations in children. However, in adults, data regarding the response of visfatin to weight loss are contradictory and mainly relate to diabetic or severely obese patients. Both decreases and increases in visfatin concentration have been reported in morbidly obese subjects after surgery [69–71]. Similarly, exercise was reported to lower visfatin in patients with type I diabetes [52], in patients at the early onset of type 2 diabetes [72], in healthy but obese patients [49] or increase visfatin concentration or expression in healthy male subjects [73].

Jürimäe et al. [9] found that plasma visfatin concentration was positively related to insulin resistance and overall adiposity markers in physically active girls. At the same time, adiponectin was negatively related to fat mass and central adiposity values, and positively related to FFM, suggesting a contribution of visfatin and adiponectin to insulin resistance and FFM, respectively. Further, Jürimäe et al. [9] showed that visfatin, but not adiponectin or leptin, was one of the independent variables to characterize HOMA in physically active girls. Given that insulin sensitivity has been reported to improve with exercise training [63], the positive association between plasma visfatin and insulin resistance could indicate that visfatin may be involved in the regulation of insulin sensitivity and a decreased visfatin concentration may have exerted a positive effect on insulin sensitivity.

Frydelund-Larsen et al. [73] found that plasma visfatin concentrations were not altered by 3 h of cycle ergometer test at 60% of VO_{2max}, whereas mRNA expression of this cytokine in abdominal subcutaneous adipose tissue increased but it was not increased in skeletal muscle. In contrast, Jürimäe et al. [74] showed that visfatin decreased in male rowers after 2 h of rowing at individual anaerobic threshold, a significantly higher intensity than in the study by Frydelund-Larsen et al. [73]. Therefore, it can be suggested that in healthy subjects visfatin levels may decrease if the energy expenditure is high enough. This can be further supported by the fact that in contrast to cycling, where only leg muscles are used, rowing is a whole-body exercise providing a greater overall stress to the organism.

To the best of our knowledge, no studies have assessed the effect of acute or chronic exercise on visfatin concentration in children or adolescents and it is difficult to make assumptions from studies undertaken in adults. However, we suggest that in controlled conditions, decreases in visfatin levels can be obtained in obese children with long-term exercise interventions. However, further research is required before definitive conclusions can be made.

Conclusions and Suggestions for Further Studies

There is strong support in the literature for the protective role of adiponectin in the development of obesity-related disorders and the metabolic syndrome. However, it appears that adiponectin may have a greater protective role in obese compared to lean individuals [31]. Studies on the regulation of visfatin have more often yielded contradictory results. Differences in sample size, study population, physical activity level and genetic background might explain the different findings. Furthermore, Körner et al. [75] found that the three currently available visfatin immunoassays lead to significant discrepancies in the qualitative and quantitative detection of visfatin in humans. In their review, Sommer et al. [53] further suggested it is unlikely that visfatin will be a useful biomarker for different components of the metabolic syndrome, including visceral obesity, due to the lack of association between visfatin expression in adipose tissue and circulating visfatin on the one hand, and parameters of obesity and insulin resistance on the other. However, it has to be pointed out that no highly controlled prospective trials have been published to investigate the potential of visfatin as a marker of metabolic and cardiovascular disease. To date, the majority of the studies have had contrary results regarding the effect of exercise on adiponectin and visfatin concentrations which does not indicate the effectiveness of exercise but rather, other uncontrolled factors.

Exercise has an impact on the adipose tissue where adiponectin and visfatin are mostly secreted. However, changes in these cytokines depends on several factors including body composition, sex, age, current disease, physical activity level, type of exercise/intervention, etc. In order to clearly investigate the effects of exercise or physical activity on adiponectin and visfatin, all of these factors should be considered in future studies.

References

1 Roemmich JN, Clark P, Lusk M, Friel A: Pubertal alterations in growth and body composition: pubertal insulin resistance – relationship to adiposity, body fat distribution and hormone release. In J Obes 2002;26:701–709.

2 Sharma AM, Chetty VT: Obesity, hypertension and insulin resistance. Acta Diabetol 2005;42:3–8.

3 Nemet D, Wang P, Funahashi T, Matsuzawa Y, Tanaka S, Engelman L, Cooper DM: Adipocytokines, body composition, and fitness in children. Pediatr Res 2003;53:148–152.

4 Fontana L, Eagon JC, Trujillo ME, Scherer PE, Klein S: Visceral fat adipokine secretion is associated with systemic inflammation in obese humans. Diabetes 2007;56:1010–1013.

5 Jin H, Jiang B, Tang J, Lu W, Wang W, Zhou L, Shang W, Li F, Ma Q, Yang Y, Chen M, Segawa K, Tanaka M, Kishimoto K, Matsuki Y, Murakami M, Ichisaka T, Murakami H, Watanabe E, Takagi T, Akiyoshi M, Ohtsubo T, Kihara S, Yamashita S, Makishima M, Funahashi T, Yamanaka S, Hiramatsu R, Matsuzawa Y, Shimomura I: Serum visfatin concentrations in obese adolescents and its correlates with age and high-density lipoprotein cholesterol. Diabetes Res Clin Pract 2008;79:412–418.

6 Pomerants T, Tillmann V, Karelson K, Jürimäe J, Jürimäe T: Ghrelin response to acute aerobic exercise in boys at different stages of puberty. Horm Metab Res 2006;38:752–757.

7 Araki S, Dobashi K, Kubo K, Kawagoe R, Yamamoto Y, Kawada Y, Asayama K, Shiharata A: Plasma visfatin concentration as a surrogate marker for visceral fat accumulation in obese children. Obesity 2008; 16:384–388.

8 Moon Y, Kim D, Song D: Serum tumor necrosis factor-alpha levels and components of the metabolic syndrome in obese adolescents. Metabolism 2004; 53:863–867.

9 Jürimäe J, Gruodyte R, Saar M, Cicchella A, Stefanelli C, Passariello C, Maasalu K, Jürimäe T, von Duvillard SP: Plasma visfatin and adiponectin concentrations in physically active adolescent girls: relationships with insulin sensitivity and body composition variables. Eur J Appl Physiol 2010 Submitted.

10 Caprio S: Insulin resistance in childhood obesity. J Pediatr Endocrinol Metab 2002;15(suppl 1):487–492.

11 Franks PW: Obesity, inflammatory markers and cardiovascular disease: distinguishing causality from confounding. J Hum Hypert 2006;20:837–840.

12 Metcalf BS, Jeffery AN, Hosking J, Voss LD, Sattar N, Wilkin TJ: Objectively measured physical activity and its association with adiponectin and other novel metabolic markers. Diab Care 2009;32:468–473.

13 Motoshima H, Wu X, Sinha MK, Hardy VE, Rosato EL, Barbot DJ, Rosato FE, Goldstein BJ: Differential regulation of adiponectin secretion from cultured human omental and subcutaneous adipocytes: effects of insulin and rosiglitazone. J Clin Endocrinol Metab 2002;87:5662–5667.

14 Pilz S, Horejsi R, Moller R, Almer G, Scharnagl H, Stojanovic T, Dimitrova R, Weihrauch G, Borkenstein M, Maerz W, Schauenstein K, Mangge H: Early atherosclerosis in obese juveniles is associated with low serum levels of adiponectin. J Clin Endocrinol Metab 2005;90:4792–4796.

15 Yamauchi T, Kamon J, Minokoshi Y, Ito Y, Waki H, Uchida S, Yamashita S, Noda M, Kita S, Ueki K, Eto K, Akanuma Y, Froguel P, Foufelle F, Ferre P, Carling D, Kimura S, Nagai R, Kahn BB, Kadowaki T: Adiponectin stimulates glucose utilization and fatty-acid oxidation by activating AMP-activated kinase. Nat Med 2002;8:1288–1295.

16 Trujillo ME, Scherer PE: Adiponectin – journey from an adipocyte secretory protein to biomarker of the metabolic syndrome. J Intern Med 2005;257:167–175.

17 Berg AH, Scherer PE: Adipose tissue, inflammation, and cardiovascular disease. Circ Res 2005;96:939–949.

18 Simpson KA, Fiatorne Singh MA: Effects of exercise on adiponectin: a systematic review. Obesity 2008; 16:241–256.

19 Arita Y, Kihara S, Ouchi N, Takahashi M, Maeda K, Miyagawa J, Hotta K, Shimomura I, Nakamura T, Miyaoka K, Kuriyama H, Nishida M, Yamashita S, Okubo K, Matsubara K, Muraguchi M, Ohmoto Y, Funahashi T, Matsuzawa Y: Paradoxical decrease of an adipose specific protein adiponectin, in obesity. Biochem Biophys Res Commun 1999;257:79–83.

20 Spranger J, Kroke A, Mohlig M, Bergmann MM, Ristow M, Boeing H, Pfeiffer AF: Adiponectin and protection against type 2 diabetes mellitus. Lancet 2003;361:226–228.

21 Ouchi N, Kihara S, Arita Y, Okamoto Y, Maeda K, Kuriyama H, Hotta K, Nishida M, Takahashi M, Muraguchi M, Ohmoto Y, Nakamura T, Yamashita S, Funahashi T, Matsuzawa Y: Adiponectin, an adipocyte-derived plasma protein, inhibits endothelial NF-kappaB signaling through a cAMP-dependent pathway. Circulation 2000;102:1296–1301.

22 Chen MP, Chung FM, Chang DM, Tsai JCR, Huang HF, Shin SJ, Lee YJ: Elevated plasma level of visfatin/pre-B cell colony-enhancing factor in patients with type 2 diabetes mellitus. J Clin Endocrinol Metab 2006;91:295–299.

23 Samal B, Sun Y, Stearns G, Xie C, Suggs S, McNiece I: Cloning and characterization of the cDNA encoding a novel human pre-cell colony enchancing factor. Mol Cell Biol 1994;14:1431–1437.

24 Haider DG, Holzer G, Schaller G, Weghuber D, Widhalm K, Wagner O, Kapiotis S, Wolzt M: The adipokine visfatin is markedly elevated in obese children. J Pediatr Gastroenterol Nutr 2006;43:548–549.

25 Ognjanovic S, Bao S, Yamamoto SY, Garibay-Tupas J, Samal B, Bryant-Greenwood GD: Genomic organization of the gene coding for human pre-B cell colony-enchancing factor and expression in human fetal membranes. J Mol Endocrinol 2001;26:107–117.

26 Kralisch S, Klein J, Lossner U, Bluher M, Pashke R, Stumvoll M, Fasshauer M: Interleukin 6 is a negative regulator of visfatin gene expression in 3T3-L1 adipocytes. J Endocrinol 2005;185:1–8.

27 Böttner A, Kratzsch J, Müller G, Kapellen TM, Blüher S, Keller E, Blüher M, Kiess W: Gender differences of adiponectin levels develop during the progression of puberty and are related to serum androgen levels. J Clin Endocrinol Metab 2004;89: 4053–4061.

28 Punthakee Z, Delvin EE, O'Loughlin J, Paradis G, Levy E, Platt RW, Lambert M: Adiponectin, adiposity, and insulin resistance in children and adolescents. J Clin Endorinol Metab 2006;91:2119–2125.

29 Cruz M, Garcia-Valerio Y, Gutierrez M, Medina-Navarro R, Duran G, Wacher N, Kumate J: Low adiponectin levels predict type 2 diabetes in Mexican children. Diabetes Care 2004;27:1451–1453.

30 Tsou PL, Jiang YD, Chang CC, Wei JN, Sung FC, Lin CC, Chiang CC, Tai TY, Chuang LM: Sex related differences between adiponectin and insulin resistance in schoolchildren. Diabetes Care 2004;27:308–313.

31 Rubin DA, McMurray RG, Harrell JA, Hackney AC, Thorpe DE, Haqq AM: The association between insulin resistance and cytokines in adolescents: the role of weight status and exercise. Metabolism 2008; 57:683–690.

32 Jürimäe J, Purge P, Jürimäe T: Adiponectin and stress hormone responses to maximal sculling after volume-extended training season in elite rowers. Metabolism 2006;55:13–19.

33 Stefan N, Bunt JC, Salbe AD, Funahashi T, Matsuzawa Y, Tataranni PA: Plasma adiponectin concentrations in children: relationships with obesity and insulinemia. J Clin Endorinol Metab 2002;87: 4652–4656.

34 Ong KK, Frystyk J, Flyvbjerg A, Petry CJ, Ness A, Dunger DB: Sex-discordant associations with adiponectin levels and lipid profiles in children. Diabetes 2006;55:1337–1341.

35 Weyer C, Funahashi T, Tanaka S, Hotta K, Matsuzawa Y, Pratley RE, Tataranni PA: Hypoadiponectinemia in obesity and type 2 diabetes: close association with insulin resistance and hyperinsulinemia. J Clin Endocrinol Metab 2001;86:1930–1935.

36 Yamauchi M, Kamon J, Waki H: The fat derived hormone adiponectin reverses insulin resistance associated with both lipoathropy and obesity. Nat Med 2001;7:941–946.

37 Vendrell J, Broch M, Villarrasa N, Molina A, Gómez JM, Gutiérrez C, Simón I, Soler I, Soler J, Richart C: Resistin, adiponectin, ghrelin, leptin, and proinflammatory cytokines: relationships in obesity. Obes Res 2004;12:962–971.

38 Maeda N, Shimomura I, Kishida K, Nishizawa H, Matsuda M, Nagaretani H, Furuyama N, Kondo H, Takahashi M, Arita Y, Komuro R, Ouchi N, Kihara S, Tochino Y, Okutomi K, Horie M, Takeda S, Aoyama T, Funahashi T, Matsuzawa Y: Diet-induced insulin resistance in mice lacking adiponectin/ACRP30. Nat Med 2002;8:731–737.

39 Kern PA, Di Gregorio GB, Lu T, Rassouli N, Ranganathan G: Adiponectin expression from human adipose tissue: relationships to obesity insulin resistance, and tumor necrosis factor-alpha expression. Diabetes 2003;52:1779–1785.

40 Hotta K, Funahashi T, Arita Y, Takahashi M, Matsuda M, Okamoto Y, Iwahashi H, Kuriyama H, Ouchi N, Maeda K, Nishida M, Kihara S, Sakai N, Nakajima T, Hasegawa K, Muraguchi M, Ohmoto Y, Nakamura T, Yamashita S, Hanafusa T, Matsuzawa Y: Plasma concentrations of a novel, adipose-specific protein, adiponectin, in type 2 diabetic patients. Arterioscler Thromb Vasc Biol 2000;20:1595–1599.

41 Monzillo LU, Hamdy OA, Horton ES, Ledbury S, Mullooly C, Jarema C, Porter S, Ovalle K, Moussa A, Mantzorost CS: Effect of lifestyle modification on adipokine levels in obese subjects with insulin resistance. Obes Res 2003;11:1048–1054.

42 Huang KC, Lue BH, Yen RF, Shen CG, Ho SR, Tai TY, Yang WS: Plasma adiponectin levels and metabolic factors in nondiabetic adolescents. Obes Res 2004;12:119–124.

43 Sethi JK, Vidal-Puig A: Visfatin: the missing link between intra-abdominal obesity and diabetes? Trends Mol Med 2005;11:344–347.

44 Davutoglu M, Ozkaya M, Guler E, Garipardic M, Gursoy H, Karabiber H, Kilmc M: Plasma visfatin concentrations in childhood obesity: relationships to insulin resistance and anthropometic indices. Swiss Med Wkly 2009;139:22–27.

45 Berndt J, Klöting N, Kralisch S, Kovacs P, Fasshauer M, Schön MR, Sumvoll M, Blüher M: Plasma visfatin concentration and fat depot-specific mRNA expression in humans. Diabetes 2005;54:2911–2916.

46 Pagano C, Pilon C, Olivieri M, Mason P, Fabris R, Milan G, Rossato M, Federspil G, Vettor R: Reduced plasma visfatin/pre-B cell colony-enchancing factor in obesity is not related to insulin resistance in humans. J Clin Endocrinol Metab 2006;91:3165–3170.

47 Varma V, Yao-Borengasser A, Rasouli N, Bodles AM, Phanavanh B, Lee MI, Starks T, Kern LM, Spencer HJ, McGehee RE Jr, Fried SK, Kern PA: Human visfatin expression: relationships to insulin sensitivity, intramyocellular lipids, and inflammation. J Clin Endocrinol Metab 2007;92:666–672.

48 Fernandez-Real JM, Moreno JM, Chico B, Lopez-Bermejo A, Ricart W: Circulating visfatin is associated with parameters of iron metabolism in subjects with altered glucose tolerance. Diabetes Care 2007; 30:616–621.
49 Choi KM, Kim JH, Cho GJ, Baik SH, Park HS, Kim SM: Effect of exercise training on plasma visfatin and eotaxin levels. Eur J Endocrinol 2007;157:437–442.
50 Oki K, Yamane K, Kamei N, Nojima H, Kohno N: Circulating visfatin level is correlated with inflammation, but not with insulin resistance. Clin Endocrinol 2007;67:796–800.
51 Chen CC, Li TC, Li CI, Liu CS, Lin WY, Wu MT, Lai MM, Lin TC: The relationship between visfatin levels and anthropometric and metabolic parameters: association with cholesterol levels in women. Metabol Clin Exp 2007;56:1216–1260.
52 Haider DG, Pleiner J, Francesconi M, Wiesinger GF, Müller M, Wolzt M: Exercise training lowers plasma visfatin concentrations in patients with type 1 diabetes. J Clin Endocrinol Metab 2006;91:4702–4704.
53 Sommer G, Garten A, Petzold S, Beck-Sickinger AG, Blüher M, Stumvoll M, Fasshauer M: Visfatin/PBEF/Nampt: structure, regulation and potential function of a novel adipokine. Clin Sci 2008;115:12–23.
54 Jian WX, Luo TH, Gu YY, Zhang HL, Zheng S, Dai M, Han JF, Zhao Y, Li G, Luo M: The visfatin gene is associated with glucose and lipid metabolism in a Chinese population. Diabet Med 2006;23:967–973.
55 Yokoyama H, Emoto M, Araki T, Fujiwara S, Motoyama K, Morioka T, Koyama H, Shoji T, Okuno Y, Nishizava Y: Effect of aerobic exercise on plasma adiponectin levels and insulin resistance in type 2 diabetes. Diabetes Care 2004;27:1756–1758.
56 Nemet D, Oh Y, Kim H, Hill M, Cooper DM: Effect of intense exercise on inflammatory cytokines and growth mediators in adolescent boys. Pediatrics 2002;67:796–800.
57 Platat C, Wagner A, Klumpp T, Schweitzer B, Simon C: Relationships of physical activity with metabolic syndrome features and low-grade inflammation in adolescents. Diabetology 2006;49:2078–2085.
58 Balagopal P, George D, Yarandi H, Funanage V, Bayne E: Reversal of obesity-related hypoadiponectinemia by lifestyle intervention: a controlled, randomized study in obese adolescents. J Clin Endocrinol Metab 2005;90:6192–6197.
59 Fatouros IG, Tournis S, Leontsini D, Jamurtas AZ, Sxina M, Thomakos P, Manousaki M, Douroudos I, Taxildaris K, Mitrakou A: Leptin and adiponectin responses in overweight inactive elderly following resistance training and detraining are intensity related. J Clin Endocrinol Metab 2005;90:5970–5977.
60 Jürimäe J, Purge P, Jürimäe T: Adiponectin is altered after maximal exercise in highly trained rowers. Eur J Appl Physiol 2005;93:502–505.
61 Takanami Y, Kawai Y, Kinoshita F, Mobara O, Shimotsitsu T: Aerobic exercise training increases adipocyte-derived anti-diabetic, anti-atherogenic protein, adiponectin. Diabetes 2002;51:61.
62 Yatagai T, Nishida Y, Nagasaka S, Nakamura T, Tokuyama K, Shindo M, Tanaka H, Ishibashi S: Relationship between exercise training-induced increase in insulin sensitivity and adiponectinemia in healthy men. Endocrinol J 2003;50:233–238.
63 Hulver MW, Zheng D, Tanner CJ, Houmard JA, Kraus WE, Slentz S, Sinha MK, Pories WJ, MacDonald KG, Dohm GI: Adiponectin is not altered with exercise training despite enchanced insulin action. Am J Physiol 2002;283:861–865.
64 Nassis GP, Papantakou K, Skenderi K, Triandafillopoulou M, Kavouras SA, Yannakoulia M, Chrousos GP, Sidossis LS: Aerobic exercise training improves insulin sensitivity without changes in body weight, body fat, adiponectin, and innflammatory markers in overweight and obese girls. Metabolism 2005;54:1427–1479.
65 Ferguson MA, White LJ, McCoy S, Kim HW, Petty T, Wilsey J: Plasma adiponectin response to acute exercise in healthy subjects. Eur J Appl Physiol 2004; 91:324–329.
66 Punyadeera C, Zorenc AHG, Koopman R, McAinch AJ, Smit E, Manders R, Keizer HA, Cameron-Smith D, van Loon LJ: The effects of adipose tissue lipolysis on plasma adiponectin concentration and adiponectin receptor expression in human skeletal muscle. Eur J Endocrinol 2005;152:427–436.
67 Cambuli VM, Musiu C, Incani M, Paderi M, Serpe R, Marras V, Cossu E, Cavallo MG, Mariotti S, Loche S, Baroni MG: Assesment of adiponectin and leptin as biomarkers of positive metabolic outcomes after lifestyle intervention in overweight and obese children. J Clin Endocrinol Metab 2008;93:3051–3057.
68 Froberg K, Andresen LB: Mini review: Physical activity and fitness and its relations to cardiovascular disease risk factors in children. Int J Obes (Lond) 2005;29:34–39.
69 Haider DG, Schindler K, Schaller G, Prager G, Woltz M, Ludvik B: Increased plasma visfatin concentrations in morbidly obese subjects are reduced after gastric binding. J Clin Endocrinol Metab 2006; 91:1578–1581.
70 Manco M, Fernandez-Real JM, Equitani F, Vendrell J, Valera Mora ME, Nanni G, Tondolo V, Calvani M, Ricart W, Castagneto M, Mingrone G: Effect of massive weight loss on inflammatory adipocytokines and the innate immune system in morbidly obese women. J Clin Endocrinol Metab 2007;92:482–490.

71 Krzyzanovska K, Mittermayer F, Krugluger W, Kopp HP, Schernthaner G: Increase in visfatin after weight loss induced gastroplastic surgery. Obesity 2006;14: 1886–1889.

72 Brema I, Hatunic F, Finucane N, Burns J, Nolan J, Haider D, Woltzt M, Ludvik B: Plasma visfatin is reduced after aerobic exercise in early onset type 2 diabetes mellitus. Diabetes Obes Metab 2008;10:593–602.

73 Frydelund-Larsen L, Akerstrom T, Nielsen S, Keller P, Keller C, Pedersen BK: Visfatin mRNA expression in human subcutaneous adipose tissue is regulated by exercise. Am J Physiol Endocrinol Metab 2007; 292:24–31.

74 Jürimäe J, Rämson R, Mäestu J, Purge P, Jürimäe T, Arciero PJ, von Duvillard SP: Plasma visfatin and ghrelin response to prolonged sculling in competitive male rowers. Med Sci Sports Exec 2009;41:137–143.

75 Körner A, Kratzsch J, Kiess W: Adipocytokines: leptin – the classical, resistin – the controversial, adiponectin – the promising, and more to come. Pr Res Clin Endorinol Metab 2005;19:525–546.

Jarek Mäestu, PhD
Institute of Sport Pedagogy and Coaching Sciences
Centre for Behavioral and Health Sciences, University of Tartu
Jakobi 5, 51014 Tartu (Estonia)
Tel. +372 7 375 372, Fax +372 7 375 373, E-Mail Jarek.Maestu@ut.ee

Jürimäe J, Hills AP, Jürimäe T (eds): Cytokines, Growth Mediators and Physical Activity in Children during Puberty.
Med Sport Sci. Basel, Karger, 2010, vol 55, pp 69–81

Ghrelin and Obestatin Concentrations during Puberty: Relationships with Adiposity, Nutrition and Physical Activity

N.A. King[a] · C.H. Gibbons[b] · C. Martins[c]

[a]Institute of Health and Biomedical Innovation, Queensland University of Technology, Brisbane, Australia; [b]Institute of Psychological Sciences, University of Leeds, Leeds, UK; [c]Obesity Research Center, Institute of Cancer and Molecular Medicine, Faculty of Medicine, Norwegian University of Science and Technology, Trondheim, Norway

Abstract

Ghrelin and obestatin are two peptides associated with appetite control and the regulation of energy balance in adults. It is intuitive that they have an important role in growth and development during puberty. Therefore, it is acknowledged that these peptides, in addition to others, form part of the substrate underlying energy homeostasis which in turn will contribute to body weight regulation and could explain changes in energy balance during puberty. Both peptides originate from the stomach; hence, it is intuitive that they are involved in generating signals from tissue stores which influence food intake. This could be manifested via alterations in the drive to eat (i.e. hunger), eating behaviors and appetite regulation. Furthermore, there is some evidence that these peptides might also be associated with physical activity behaviors and metabolism. Anecdotally, children and adolescents experience behavioral and metabolic changes during growth and development which will be associated with physiological changes.

This chapter outlines how these two peptides, independently and collectively, are associated with changes in energy balance during puberty by focusing on behavioral factors; eating and physical activity. Ghrelin and obestatin exert a marked effect on the motivation to eat and food intake and are modulated during puberty by habitual physical activity levels. Diurnal profiles of ghrelin are strongly associated with changes in energy balance, increasing with weight reduction and decreasing with weight gain. There is some indication that there are gender differences. The conclusions concerning the role of obestatin are less clear, mainly due to the limited number of studies.

Ghrelin during Puberty: Relationships with Adiposity, Nutrition and Physical Activity

Introduction

Ghrelin, a peptide of 28 amino acids predominantly produced in the stomach [1], has contributed considerably to the understanding of appetite control, energy balance (EB) and growth in recent years. In addition to its growth hormone-releasing properties [2], ghrelin has been found to promote positive EB by increasing appetite and food intake [3, 4] and reducing fat oxidation and energy expenditure in rodents [5]. The acylation of ghrelin is thought to be essential for ghrelin to exert its orexigenic effects at the hypothalamic level [6, 7]. Ghrelin reflects both acute and chronic feeding states in humans [1]. Its concentrations increase with fasting and quickly decline after a meal [1] and have been shown to be associated with premeal hunger and meal initiation [8]. Moreover, ghrelin concentrations are significantly reduced in obese subjects [9] and markedly elevated in patients with anorexia nervosa [1], likely as an adaptive mechanism.

Cross-sectional studies conducted in healthy children and adolescents have shown that ghrelin levels peak in early postnatal life (around 2 years of age) [10] and then gradually decrease during childhood and adolescence until the end of puberty [10–12]. A significant negative correlation has been described between fasting ghrelin plasma levels and age [11, 13–16] and pubertal development [11, 15, 17]. However, the changes experienced during puberty seem to be less pronounced in girls compared with boys [11]. Ghrelin plasma levels have also been shown to be significantly higher in girls compared with boys [16, 18]. A pharmacological increase in sex hormones in short peripubertal children has been shown to lead to a marked decline in circulating plasma levels of ghrelin in boys but not in girls [19], suggesting that sex hormones modulate ghrelin secretion and are responsible for the distinct ghrelin profile during puberty in boys and girls. Some studies, however, report no difference in ghrelin plasma levels between girls and boys [12, 20–23] or children and adults [20, 24], and no reduction in fasting ghrelin plasma levels with increasing age [21] or sexual development [20, 21]. A small sample size [12, 20, 24], and a narrow range of pubertal development and age (7–11 years) [20] are likely to have contributed to the negative results observed in some of these studies.

Anecdotally, puberty tends to be characterized by an increase in the desire to eat, food intake and body weight. Paradoxically, this period is associated with a reduction in ghrelin plasma levels. It has been suggested that there could be an increased sensitivity to the orexigenic properties of this hormone during puberty, in order to sustain growth during this period [11].

Relationship with Adiposity

Similar to adults [1, 9], fasting total ghrelin (TG) plasma levels are significantly lower in obese children and adolescents [12, 15, 20, 21, 23, 25–29], and significantly higher in adolescents with anorexic nervosa [12, 28, 30, 31], compared with normal-weight (NW) controls, matched for age and puberty status. The ratio of ghrelin:obestatin has also been reported to be significantly lower in obese compared with NW children [21, 26]. Obese children [15, 32] and adolescents [15, 33] are characterized by lower AG plasma levels compared with NW controls. However, the AG:TG ratio was markedly higher in obese children and adolescents compared with NW controls (43 vs. 28%) [15], suggesting that even though obese children present with low TG plasma levels, their 'relative' orexigenic drive to eat is not necessarily lower than in NW children.

Consistent with these patterns, there is a negative relationship between fasting TG plasma levels and body mass index (BMI) [13, 14, 17, 18, 22, 23, 27–29, 34, 35], BMI standard deviation scores (SDS) [11, 21, 26], weight [17, 18, 21, 35, 36], weight SDS [11, 17], absolute [27, 35, 37] or relative fat mass [18, 23, 26, 27, 36, 38], as well as with other measures of adiposity such as waist circumference [14, 18], hip circumference [18], waist/hip ratio [18] and waist/height ratio [14]. Ghrelin has also been described to be negatively correlated with fat-free mass (FFM) in active [34, 35] and inactive boys [17, 35], but not in adolescent girls with different levels of physical activity (PA) [37]. The association between ghrelin and height remains ambiguous with some studies reporting a negative association [17, 18, 36] and others not [11] or a correlation in active, but not in inactive boys [35].

Fasting TG plasma levels are inversely correlated with insulin resistance [22, 23] and fasting insulin plasma levels in children in most [13, 16, 17, 20–23, 27, 36, 39], but not all studies [12, 24, 29], or only in boys but not in girls [18]. Moreover, this association seems to be independent of BMI [23, 27] and fat mass [27]. The negative association between TG and weight and adiposity no longer exists when insulin plasma levels are controlled for [36].

Collectively, these findings suggest that the low levels of ghrelin observed in obese children are a manifestation of the insulin resistance characteristic of obesity, which has an inhibitory effect on ghrelin secretion, rather than excess weight in itself [22, 27]. Stylianou et al. [23], however, reported significantly lower ghrelin plasma levels in obese adolescents with and without insulin resistance, compared with NW controls, matched for age and gender, despite significantly lower ghrelin levels in obese insulin resistant adolescents compared with those without insulin resistance. This suggests that although insulin resistance plays an important role in ghrelin secretion, other factors also contribute to the low ghrelin levels in obese children and adolescents.

Data concerning the association between changes in ghrelin plasma levels and weight loss in children and adolescents are equivocal. A 1-year weight loss

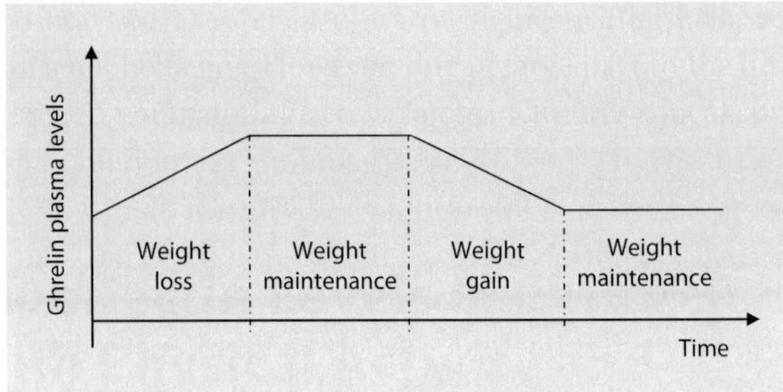

Fig. 1. Proposed temporal profile of ghrelin response to changes in body weight.

intervention in obese children and adolescents, involving PA, behavioral education and dietary modification had no impact on fasting TG plasma levels [25, 26], increased fasting obestatin and induced a slight decrease in the ghrelin/obestatin ratio [26], despite a significant reduction in fasting insulin plasma levels, and improvement in insulin sensitivity [25, 26]. An energy-restricted diet in prepubertal obese children leading to a 25% and 50% reduction in BMI SD at 6 and 12 months, respectively, was, however, associated with a significant increase in fasting TG plasma levels [12]. However, this reduction in BMI SD is considerably greater than that observed in the previous studies [25, 26]. On the other hand, a 25% and 50% recuperation of BMI SD in anorexic adolescents during a nutrition programme, achieved at 2 months and 1 year, respectively, was associated with a significant reduction in TG plasma levels [12].

Weight loss after a 1-month weight loss camp was associated with a significant increase in fasting TG, obestatin and the ghrelin/obestatin ratio in obese children and these changes were correlated with improvements in insulin sensitivity [21]. Moreover, a short-term energy restriction combined with PA (10 days) in obese children and adolescents, induced a significant reduction in BMI and was associated with an increase in fasting TG levels [40]. Diet-induced weight loss over 6 weeks in obese children has also been shown to increase total daily (area under the curve, AUC) ghrelin in response to an oral glucose tolerance test (OGTT) and this increase correlated positively with insulin sensitivity at baseline and with the magnitude of improvement in insulin sensitivity observed over time [41].

Kelishadi et al. [14] demonstrated that ghrelin increases significantly in response to weight loss induced either by dietary restriction or increased PA for 6 months in prepubertal children, but it returned to baseline levels during weight stabilization [14]. Therefore, although ghrelin automatically increases during weight loss, it returns to baseline levels with sustained weight maintenance [42], suggesting that although ghrelin may respond to acute (episodic) changes in EB and body weight it is unlikely to regulate long-term (tonic) EB (fig. 1).

Relationship with Nutrition

A diurnal variation in ghrelin secretion has been described in NW girls, with ghrelin increasing during the preprandial state and decreasing during the postprandial state. However, in obese girls ghrelin levels fail to increase in response to prolonged fasting [43]. Data concerning the impact of food intake on ghrelin plasma levels in children and adolescents are mixed. Lomenick et al. [44] reported no suppression of TG after a mixed composition breakfast or a pre-prandial rise before lunch, in either NW or overweight children. Similar results were described by Bellone et al. [24] in prepubertal NW children after a light breakfast. Misra et al. [33] also showed no suppression of AG after meals high in fat, protein or carbohydrate in either NW or obese adolescent girls. Surprisingly, there was an increase in AG levels after the high-carbohydrate meal in obese adolescent girls.

Stock et al. [28] reported a significant suppression of TG after a mixed meal in NW, obese and anorexic adolescents, with no difference in percent maximum decrease between groups, despite a smaller absolute reduction in the obese group [28]. A significant suppression of TG levels after a mixed composition meal has also been reported in prepubertal overweight boys [45, 46] and in NW and obese prepubertal children [16]. A significant suppression of TG plasma levels has also been reported after an OGTT in NW [27, 29, 30, 41] and obese children [27, 29, 41, 47] and anorexic adolescent girls [30], with no differences in the extent of ghrelin suppression between groups [27, 29, 30, 47]. Lanyi et al. [32] showed a significant suppression of AG plasma levels after an OGTT in NW, but not in obese children who experienced an increase in AG plasma levels at 120 min postprandially.

Variations in the macronutrient composition of the test meal, sampling time and frequency, children's characteristics (e.g. gender and pubertal status), and sample size between studies are likely to contribute to the lack of consistency among studies regarding the impact of feeding on ghrelin plasma levels during puberty. It has been suggested that a minimum amount of carbohydrate, sufficient to increase glucose and insulin plasma levels, is required to induce a significant suppression in ghrelin during the postprandial state [29].

Relationship with Physical Activity

Ghrelin plasma levels throughout puberty seem to be modulated by PA levels. While fasting TG plasma levels fall throughout puberty in inactive boys [11, 17, 35], they remain unchanged [35] or decrease only until the onset of puberty, but not with advancing puberty stages in physically active boys [34]. Jürimäe et al. [35] reported significantly higher fasting TG plasma levels in physically active boys in Tanner stage II and above compared with inactive controls, matched for age and BMI, but not in Tanner stage I (prepubertal) [35]. This is in accordance with another study showing higher TG plasma levels in physically active adolescent girls compared with physically inactive girls with different pubertal maturation (Tanner stage II up to V) [37]. High PA levels prevent the typical fall in TG plasma levels observed during puberty. This could be an adaptive mechanism which is designed to stimulate appetite and food intake in the presence of high activity-induced energy expenditure in an attempt to prevent weight loss and facilitate growth.

Ghrelin plasma levels have also been reported to be positively correlated with weekly exercise (frequency of exercise/week), but only marginally with VO_{2max}, in adolescent girls [38]. This may suggest that the impact of regular exercise on ghrelin plasma levels is achieved through disturbances in EB (by increasing energy expenditure and thus creating an energy deficit), rather than by its impact on cardiovascular fitness. Later studies have reported controversial results regarding the association between fitness and ghrelin plasma levels. VO_{2max} was found to be negatively correlated with ghrelin in inactive [34, 35], but not in active boys [35], and to be positively correlated in active and inactive adolescent girls [37]. It is possible that the association between fitness and ghrelin levels is modulated by gender, with only girls experiencing an increase in ghrelin concentration with increasing fitness levels. Sex hormones are likely to be involved in this gender difference, since it has been shown that they modulate ghrelin secretion [19].

Obestatin during Puberty: Relationships with Adiposity, Nutrition and Physical Activity

Introduction

The previous section explained how ghrelin is related to growth, adiposity, nutrition and physical activity. Given that ghrelin is derived by post-translational cleavage from a prepropeptide of 117 residues, another peptide was discovered in 2005; obestatin [48]. This hormone is a 23-amino acid peptide whose biological activity is dependent on the amidation at its carboxyl-terminus [49] (fig. 2). Initial studies in rodents found obestatin to exert a different effect to ghrelin by having an anorexigenic action [48]. Treatment with ghrelin in these rodents resulted in an increase in body weight, whilst obestatin suppressed body-weight gain when given at similar doses. Obestatin also led to decreased jejunal contractile activity which may induce a central satiety response via an afferent vagus signal [48]. The initial receptor for obestatin was thought to be GPR39 which belongs to the ghrelin receptor subfamily and is expressed in the jejunum, duodenum, stomach [48] and adipose tissue [50] suggesting obestatin has a role in energy homeostasis; however, other studies have been unable to replicate these findings [51, 52]. Likewise, studies have been unable to replicate the original finding that obestatin has a role in food intake and body weight regulation [53–55]. Reproducing the initial findings regarding obestatin

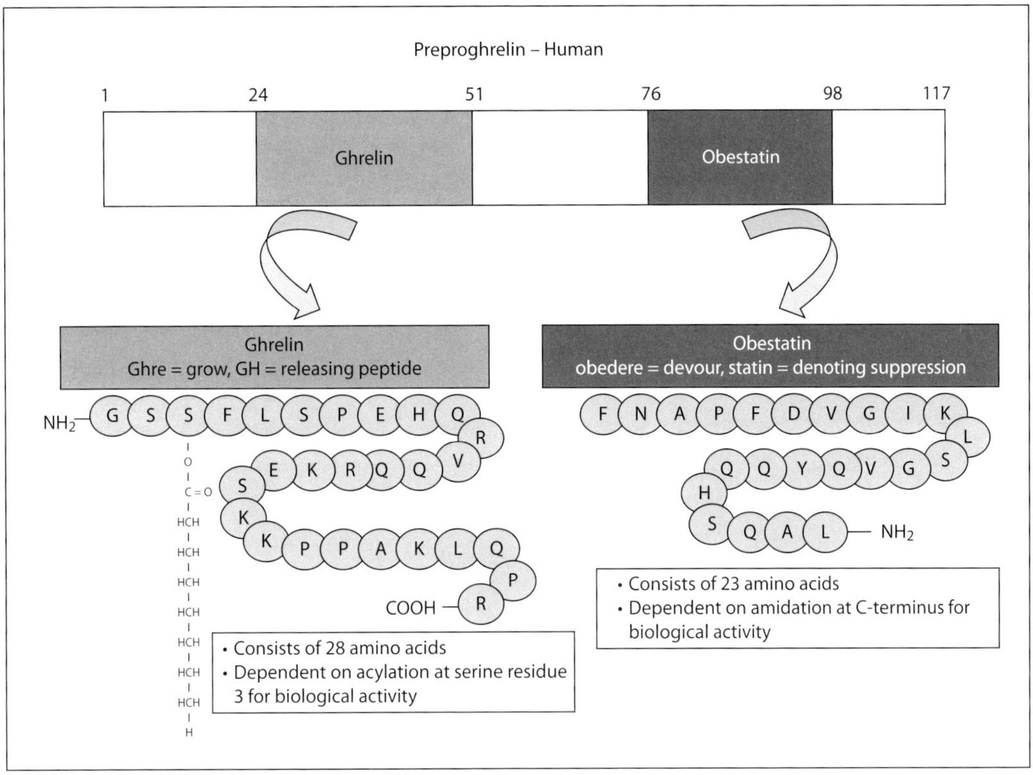

Fig. 2. The chemical structures of ghrelin and obestatin.

is controversial and may be due to dosage, route or different animal models [55]. Although ghrelin and obestatin are derived from the same protein, they have different receptors and are thought to exert opposing physiological actions which highlights that monitoring ghrelin transcript levels does not predict the secretion of obestatin [48].

There is a considerable lack of data in human subjects. To the best of our knowledge only two studies to date have investigated obestatin in both NW and obese children [56, 57]. Currently, data do not exist which track obestatin levels during the developing life stages. Obestatin levels are thought to be independent of age [58]. No differences were found between girls and boys or between prepubertal children and pubertal children with regards to obestatin levels [56]. However, in a different study there was a significant difference between boys and girls; boys had higher levels, but there was no association between obestatin and sexual development [57]. Due to the lack of studies, it is difficult to formulate a reliable argument regarding obestatin levels during puberty (see table 1 for a summary).

Table 1. States in which obestatin level may differ during puberty

Low obestatin concentration	High obestatin concentration
Girls	boys
Obesity	normal weight

Relationship with Adiposity

Whilst ghrelin tends to be lower in the obese, a possible adaptation to long-term energy balance [59], it still exhibits similar orexigenic effects as in the lean state [60]. This leads to the concept that the equilibrium between ghrelin and obestatin is important for energy homeostasis and body weight regulation [61]. In obese children, obestatin has been reported to be both significantly higher [56] and slightly lower [57] compared to NW, whilst both ghrelin and the ghrelin:obestatin ratio were significantly lower compared to the NW groups [56, 57]. Reports of the effect of weight loss on the circulating levels of obestatin are limited. Weight loss in obese children resulted in increased obestatin levels [56, 57]. In these children, ghrelin concentrations either did not change [56] or increased significantly [57], and the ratio of ghrelin:obestatin showed either a tendency to decrease [56] or increase significantly [57] after weight loss. Neither ghrelin nor obestatin changed in the children who did not lose weight (fig. 3). The children who lost substantial weight were found to have significantly lower obestatin levels and significantly higher ghrelin:obestatin ratios at baseline compared to those that did not lose weight, but their obestatin levels were still significantly higher and ghrelin significantly lower at baseline compared to NW controls [56]. These findings suggest that obestatin levels may be lowered in childhood obesity and then show a tendency to return to 'normal' values in response to weight loss and therefore might play a role in the mechanism of obesity. The opposing findings between the two studies may reflect methodological differences, gender distribution differences and sample size issues.

Relationship with Nutrition

Obestatin is secreted in a pulsatile manner and displays an ultradian rhythm in rodents, similar to that of ghrelin and growth hormone secretion but with a lower number of episodes [62]. The same study in rodents also showed that obestatin levels are lowered during fasting, whilst inhibiting both food intake and gastrointestinal activity [62], yet the mechanism by which food intake is altered is, as yet, unknown. In adults, both ghrelin and obestatin significantly decrease in response to food intake.

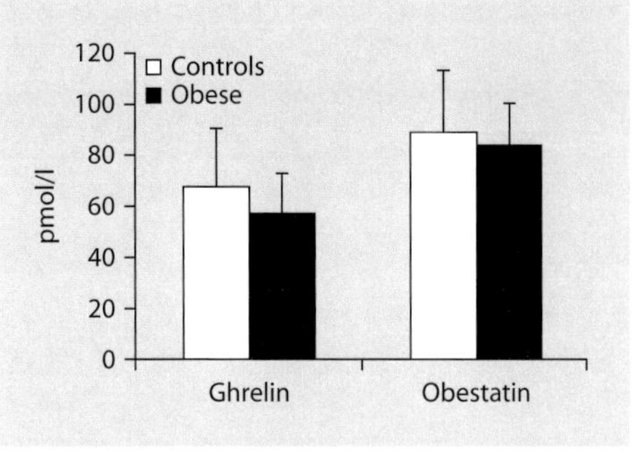

Fig. 3. Fasting ghrelin and obestatin levels in obese and lean (control) children.

Ghrelin and obestatin levels were significantly lower in the obese group compared to the lean groups both pre- and postprandially. However, the obese group had a significantly higher ghrelin:obestatin ratio than the lean group preprandially but this was not seen in the postprandial period [61]. This suggests that the balance between these peptides might enhance food intake in obese people.

A recent study investigated the effect of a high-carbohydrate breakfast on postprandial plasma obestatin and TG, AG and DG in NW women [63]. The data demonstrated that postprandial responses of AG were significantly suppressed at 30 min post-breakfast whilst obestatin, TG and DG were significantly reduced for at least 150 min post-breakfast. There was no significant change in the ghrelin:obestatin ratio during the postprandial period. The authors claim that the positive relationship between obestatin and TG suggests that they could influence food intake in a similar direction, which is further substantiated by a positive correlation between obestatin and NPY. These findings are in juxtaposition to the initial anorexigenic findings in rodents [48].

There are no studies to date regarding obestatin and food intake during the pubertal years which highlights the need for further investigation in this area and population.

Relationship with Physical Activity

Since exercise has been found to cause significant changes in ghrelin levels, it has been hypothesized that obestatin may also be altered; however, research in this area is limited. To our knowledge no studies have investigated exercise per se on obestatin levels during puberty. One study in obese rats and acute exercise showed no changes in ghrelin or obestatin, but 8 weeks of exercise revealed it was ghrelin and not obestatin that caused exercise-induced reduction in appetite [64]. An exercise intervention study which involved a sprint schedule for 60 min/day for 6 consecutive days using female adults tracked the changes in obestatin at pre-24 h, post-24 h, post-48 h, and post-7 days. No changes in obestatin were seen at any of the time-points [65]. It is

Table 2. Conditions associated with low or high ghrelin plasma levels during puberty

Low ghrelin concentration	High ghrelin concentration
Obesity	anorexia
Weight gain	weight loss
Insulin resistance	high physical activity levels

possible that since obestatin is linked to energy balance that weight loss is needed to induce a change in this peptide; however, this is yet to be confirmed.

Conclusions and Future Directions

Ghrelin levels decrease during puberty and are a good marker of nutritional status, with lower levels in obese and higher levels in underweight children and adolescents. Plasma levels of ghrelin respond quickly to changes in EB, increasing with weight reduction and decreasing with weight gain, although these changes may be transitory and levels can return to baseline after weight stabilization. There is some evidence for an altered pattern of plasma ghrelin in the postprandial state in obese compared with NW children, but the results are controversial. Low fasting levels of ghrelin in obese children and altered (lower) ghrelin suppression after a meal are likely to be a manifestation of insulin resistance characteristic of this group. High PA levels during puberty seem to be associated with higher ghrelin concentrations, likely a compensatory mechanism to avoid weight loss in face of high energy requirements (for a summary of conditions associated with low and high levels of ghrelin during puberty, see table 2). It needs to be acknowledged that most of the studies measured only TG, which may or may not correlate with the AG. More studies are needed to clearly elucidate the role of TG and AG during puberty and its relationship with adiposity, nutrition and PA.

Obestatin does not appear to correlate with ghrelin. This is perhaps surprising since they are derived from the same gene, yet adds support that obestatin is a physiologically relevant peptide that should be studied in its own right. Both ghrelin and obestatin rely on posttranslational processes in order to assert their biological activity. Obestatin relies on amidation at its carboxyl-terminus, yet detection methods for differentiating between circulating amidated and nonamidated obestatin are not yet available. Obestatin has also been shown to rapidly degrade in the circulation making measurement extremely difficult. These methodological issues need to be addressed in a wide range of human populations before we can make legitimate arguments as to the function of obestatin in puberty and its possible role in the etiology of obesity.

References

1 Ariyasu H, Takaya K, Tagami T, et al: Stomach is a major source of circulating ghrelin, and feeding determines plasma ghrelin-like immunoreactivity levels in humans. J Clin Endocrinol Metab 2001;86: 4753–4758.

2 Arvat E, Maccario M, De Vito L, et al: Endocrine activities of ghrelin, a natural growth hormone secretagogue (GHS), in humans: comparison and interactions with hexarelin, a non-natural peptidyl GHS, and GH-releasing hormone. J Clin Endocrinol Metab 2001;86:1169–1174.

3 Cummings DE, Frayo RS, Marmonier C, Aubert R, Chapelot D: Plasma ghrelin levels and hunger scores in humans initiating meals voluntarily without time- and food-related cues. Am J Physiol Endocrinol Metab 2004;287:E289–E304.

4 Wren AM, Seal LJ, Cohen MA, et al: Ghrelin enhances appetite and increases food intake in humans. J Clin Endocrinol Metab 2001;86:5992–5995.

5 Tschop M, Smiley DL, Heiman ML: Ghrelin induces adiposity in rodents. Nature 2001;407:908–913.

6 Kojima M, Hosoda H, Date Y, Nakazato M, Matsuo H, Kangawa K: Ghrelin is a growth-hormone-releasing acylated peptide from stomach. Nature 1999;402:656–660.

7 Neary NM, Druce MR, Small CJ, Bloom SR: Acylated ghrelin stimulates food intake in the fed and fasted states but desacylated ghrelin has no effect. Gut 2006;55:135.

8 Cummings DE, Purnell JQ, Frayo RS, Schmidova K, Wisse BE, Weigle DS: A preprandial rise in plasma ghrelin levels suggests a role in meal initiation in humans. Diabetes 2001;50:1714–1719.

9 Tschop M, Weyer C, Tataranni PA, Devanarayan V, Ravussin E, Heiman ML: Circulating ghrelin levels are decreased in human obesity. Diabetes 2001;50: 707–709.

10 Soriano-Guillen L, Barrios V, Chowen JA, et al: Ghrelin levels from fetal life through early adulthood: relationship with endocrine and metabolic and anthropometric measures. J Pediatr 2004; 144: 30–35.

11 Whatmore AJ, Hall CM, Jones J, Westwood M, Clayton PE: Ghrelin concentrations in healthy children and adolescents. Clin Endocrinol (Oxf) 2003;59:649–654.

12 Soriano-Guillen L, Barrios V, Campos-Barros A, Argente J: Ghrelin levels in obesity and anorexia nervosa: effects of weight reduction or recuperation. J Pediatr 2004;144:36–42.

13 Haqq AM, Farooqi IS, O'Rahilly S, et al: Serum ghrelin levels are inversely correlated with body mass index, age, and insulin concentrations in normal children and are markedly increased in Prader-Willi syndrome. J Clin Endocrinol Metab 2003;88: 174–178.

14 Kelishadi R, Hashemipour M, Mohammadifard N, Alikhassy H, Adeli K: Short- and long-term relationships of serum ghrelin with changes in body composition and the metabolic syndrome in prepubescent obese children following two different weight loss programmes. Clin Endocrinol (Oxf) 2008;69: 721–729.

15 Vivenza D, Rapa A, Castellino N, et al: Ghrelin gene polymorphisms and ghrelin, insulin, IGF-1, leptin and anthropometric data in children and adolescents. Eur J Endocrinol 2004;151:127–133.

16 Gil-Campos M, Aguilera CM, Ramirez-Tortosa MC, Canete R, Gil A: Fasting and postprandial relationships among plasma leptin, ghrelin, and insulin in prepubertal obese children. Clin Nutr 2010;29:54–59.

17 Pomerants T, Tillmann V, Jürimäe J, Jürimäe T: Relationship between ghrelin and anthropometrical, body composition parameters and testosterone levels in boys at different stages of puberty. J Endocrinol Invest 2006;29:962–967.

18 Park HS, Lee K-U, Kim YS, Park CY: Relationships between fasting plasma ghrelin levels and metabolic parameters in children and adolescents. Metabolism 2005;54:925–929.

19 Lebenthal Y, Gat-Yablonski G, Shtaif B, Padoa A, Phillip M, Lazar L: Effect of sex hormone administration on circulating ghrelin levels in peripubertal children. J Clin Endocrinol Metab 2006;91:328–331.

20 Bellone S, Rapa A, Vivenza D, et al: Circulating ghrelin levels as function of gender, pubertal status and adiposity in childhood. J Clin Endocrinol Metab 2002;5:RC13-RC15.

21 Zou CC, Liang L, Wang CL, Fu JF, Zhao ZY: The change in ghrelin and obestatin levels in obese children after weight reduction. Acta Paediatr 2009;98: 159–165.

22 Zou CC, Liang L, Zhao ZY: Factors associated with fasting plasma ghrelin levels in children and adolescents. World J Gastroenterol 2008;14:790–794.

23 Stylianou C, Galli-Tsinopoulou A, Farmakiotis D, et al: Ghrelin and leptin levels in obese adolescents: relationship with body fat and insulin resistance. Hormones 2007;6:295–303.

24 Bellone S, Castellino N, Broglio F, et al: Ghrelin secretion in childhood is refractory to the inhibitory effect of feeding. J Clin Endocrinol Metab 2004; 89:1662–1665.
25 Reinehr T, Roth CL, Alexy U, Kersting M, Kiesse W, Andler W: Ghrelin levels before and after reduction of overweight due to a low-fat high-carbohydrate diet in obese children and adolescents. Int J Obes 2005;29:362–368.
26 Reinehr T, de Sousa G, Roth CL: Obestatin and ghrelin levels in obese children and adolescents before and after reduction of overweight. Clin Endocrinol (Oxf) 2008;68:304–310.
27 Bacha F, Arslanian SA: Ghrelin supression in overweight children: a manifestation of insulin resistance? J Clin Endocrinol Metab 2005;90:2725–2730.
28 Stock S, Leichner P, Wong ACK, et al: Ghrelin, peptide YY, glucose-dependent insulinotropic polypeptide, and hunger responses to a mixed meal in anorexic, obese, and control female adolescents. J Clin Endocrinol Metab 2005;90:2161–2168.
29 Baldelli R, Bellone S, Castellino N, et al: Oral glucose load inhibits circulating ghrelin levels to the same extent in normal and obese children. Clin Endocrinol (Oxf) 2006;64:255–259.
30 Misra M, Miller KK, Herzog DB, et al: Growth hormone and ghrelin responses to an oral glucose load in adolescent girls with anorexia nervosa and controls. J Clin Endocrinol Metab 2004;89:1605–1612.
31 Misra M, Miller KK, Kuo K, et al: Secretory dynamics of ghrelin in adolescent girls with anorexia nervosa and healthy adolescents. Am J Physiol Endocrinol Metab 2005;289:E373–E381.
32 Lanyi E, Csernus K, Erhardt E, et al: Plasma levels of acylated ghrelin during an oral glucose tolerance test in obese children. J Endocrinol Invest 2007;30: 133–137.
33 Misra M, Tsai PM, Mendes N, Miller KK, Klibanski A: Increased carbohydrate induced ghrelin secretion in obese vs. normal-weight adolescent girls. Obesity 2009;17:1689–1695.
34 Jürimäe J, Lätt E, Haljaste K, Purge P, Cicchella A, Jürimäe T: Influence of puberty on ghrelin and BMD in athletes. Int J Sports Med 2009;30:403–407.
35 Jürimäe J, Cicchella A, Tillmann V, et al: Effect of pubertal development and physical activity on plasma ghrelin concentration in boys. J Endocrinol Invest 2009;32:18–22.
36 Bunt JC, Salbe AD, Tschop MH, Delparigi A, Daychild P, Tataranni PA. Cross-sectional and prospective relationships of fasting plasma ghrelin concentrations with anthropometric measures in Pima Indian children. J Clin Endocrinol Metab 2003;88: 3761.
37 Jürimäe J, Cicchella A, Jürimäe T, et al: Regular physical activity influences plasma ghrelin concentration in adolescent girls. Med Sci Sports Exerc 2007;39:1736–1741.
38 Kasa-Vubu JK, Rosenthal A, Murdock EG, Welch KB: Impact of fatness, fitness, and ethnicity on the relationship of nocturnal ghrelin to 24-hour luteinizing hormone concentrations in adolescent girls. J Clin Endocrinol Metab 2007;92:3246–3252.
39 Stock S, Leichner P, Wong ACK, et al: Ghrelin, peptide YY, glucose-dependent insulinotropic polypeptide, and hunger responses to a mixed meal in anorexic, obese, and control female adolescents. J Clin Endocrinol Metab 2005;90:2161–2168.
40 Nitsche H, Nitsche M, Sudi K, et al: Ghrelin – an indicator for fat oxidation in obese children and adolescents during a weight reduction program. J Pediatr Endocrinol Metab 2007;20:719–723.
41 Krohn K, Boczan C, Otto B, et al: Regulation of ghrelin is related to estimated insulin sensitivity in obese children. Int J Obes 2006;30:1482–1487.
42 Garcia JM, Iyer D, Poston WSC, et al: Rise of plasma ghrelin with weight loss is not sustained during weight maintenance. Obesity Res 2006;14:–1716.
43 Foster CM, Barkan A, Kasa-Vubu JZ, Jaffe C: Ghrelin concentrations reflect body mass index rather than feeding status in obese girls. Pediatr Res 2007;62:731–734.
44 Lomenick JP, Clasey JL, Anderson JW: Meal-related changes in ghrelin, peptide YY, and appetite in normal weight and overweight children. Obesity 2008; 16:547–552.
45 Maffeis C, Bonadonna RC, Consolaro A, et al: Ghrelin, insulin sensitivity and postprandial glucose disposal in overweight and obese children. Eur J Endocrinol 2006;154:61–68.
46 Maffeis C, Surano MG, Cordioli S, Gasperotti S, Corradi M, Pinelli L: A high-fat vs. a moderate-fat meal in obese boys: nutrient balance, appetite, and gastrointestinal hormone changes. Obesity (Silver Spring) 2010;18:449–455.
47 Soriano-Guillen L, Barrios V, Martos G, Chowen JA, Campos-Barros A, Argente J: Effect of oral glucose administration on ghrelin levels in obese children. Eur J Endocrinol 2004;151:119–121.
48 Zhang JV, Ren P-G, Avsian-Kretchmer O, et al: Obestatin, a peptide encoded by the ghrelin gene, opposes ghrelin's effects on food intake. Science 2005;310:996–999.
49 Vicennati V, Genghini S, De Iasio R, et al: Circulating obestatin levels and the ghrelin/obestatin ratio in obese women. Eur J Endocrinol 2007;157:295–301.

50 Catalan V, Gomez-Ambrosi J, Rotellar F, et al: The obestatin receptor (GPR39) is expressed in human adipose tissue and is down-regulated in obesity-associated type 2 diabetes mellitus. Clin Endocrinol 2007;66:598–601.
51 Lauwers E, Landuyt B, Arckens L, Schoofs L, Luyten W: Obestatin does not activate orphan g protein-coupled receptor GP. Biochem Biophys Res Commun 2006;351:21–25.
52 Holst B, Egerod KL, Schild E, et al: GPR39 signaling is stimulated by zinc ions but not by obestatin. Endocrinology 2007;148:13–20.
53 Nogueiras R, Pfluger P, Tovar S, et al: Effects of obestatin on energy balance and growth hormone secretion in rodents. Endocrinology 2007;148:21–26.
54 Seoane LM, Al-Massadi O, Pazos Y, Pagotto U, Casanueva FF: Central obestatin administration does not modify either spontaneous or ghrelin-induced food intake in rats. J Endocrinol Invest 2006:29.
55 Gourcerol G, Coskun T, Craft LS, et al: Preproghrelin-derived peptide, obestatin, fails to influence food intake in lean or obese rodents. Obesity 2007;15:2643–2652.
56 Reinehr T, de Sousa G, Roth CL: Obestatin and ghrelin levels in obese children and adolescents before and after reduction of overweight. Clin Endocrinol 2008;68:304–310.
57 Zou CC, Liang L, Wang CL, Fu JF, Zhao ZY: The change in ghrelin and obestatin levels in obese children after weight reduction. Acta Paedatr 2009;98:159–165.
58 Lippl F, Erdmann J, Lichter N, et al: Relation of plasma obestatin levels to BMI, gender, age and insulin. Horm Metab Res 2008;40:806–812.
59 Tschop M, Weyer C, Tataranni PA, et al: Circulating ghrelin levels are decreased in human obesity. Diabetes 2001;50:707–709.
60 Druce MR, Wren AM, Park AJ, et al: Ghrelin increases food intake in obese as well as lean subjects. Int J Obes 2005;14:1130–1136.
61 Guo Z-F, Zheng X, Qin Y-W, et al: Circulating preprandial ghrelin to obestatin ratio is increased in human obesity. J Clin Endocrinol Metab 2007;92:1875–1880.
62 Zizzari P, Longchamps R, Epelbaum J, Bluet-Pajot MT: Obestatin partially affects ghrelin stimulation of food intake and GH secretion in rodents. Endocrinology 2007;148:1648–1653.
63 Sedlackova D, Dostalova I, Hainer V, et al: Simultaneous decrease of plasma obestatin and ghrlein after a high-carbohydrate breakfast in healthy women. Physiol Res 2008;57:S29–S37.
64 Wang J, Chen C, Wang R-Y: Influence of short- and long-term treadmill exercises on levels of ghrelin, obestatin and NPY in plasma and brain extraction of obese rats. Endocrine 2008;33:77–83.
65 Manshouri M, Ghanbari-Niaki A, Kraemer RR, Shemshaki A: Time course alterations of plasma obestatin and growth hormone levels in response to short-term anaerobic exercise training in college women. Appl Physiol Nutr Metab 2008;33:1246–1249.

Prof. Neil King
Institute of Health and Biomedical Innovation
Queensland University of Technology
Brisbane, 4059 (Australia)
Tel. +61 7 31386444, Fax +61 7 31385049, E-Mail n.king@qut.edu.au

Jürimäe J, Hills AP, Jürimäe T (eds): Cytokines, Growth Mediators and Physical Activity in Children during Puberty.
Med Sport Sci. Basel, Karger, 2010, vol 55, pp 82–102

Menstrual Irregularities and Energy Deficiency in Physically Active Women: The Role of Ghrelin, PYY and Adipocytokines

Jennifer L. Scheid · Mary Jane De Souza

Women's Health and Exercise Laboratory, Noll Laboratory, Department of Kinesiology, Penn State University, University Park, Pa., USA

Abstract

Menstrual cycle irregularities are often observed among physically active women and athletes who participate in physical activity ranging from recreational to competitive exercise training. Further, such irregularities have been casually linked to an energy deficiency where caloric intake is inadequate for exercise energy expenditure resulting in a suppressive effect on growth and reproduction. Adaptations consistent with chronic energy deficiency, including reductions in resting energy expenditure and total triiodothyronine, have been observed in exercising women with functional hypothalamic amenorrhea (FHA). Gut peptides and adipocytokines also appear to be altered in exercising women with FHA and have been hypothesized to be involved in the etiology of FHA. Ghrelin concentrations are elevated in exercising women with FHA. Interestingly, while fasting ghrelin, an orexigenic peptide, is elevated in women with FHA, PYY, an anorexigenic peptide, is paradoxically also elevated in women with anorexia nervosa and exercising women with FHA. Leptin, an adipocytokine, is also suppressed in FHA associated with exercise and anorexia. A critical leptin concentration threshold is suggested to be necessary for regular menses to occur. Ghrelin, PYY, and leptin all have the ability to cross the blood brain barrier and, in the hypothalamus, can modulate appetite and food intake, and are hypothesized to affect the hypothalamic-pituitary-ovarian axis. Future studies are needed to determine if ghrelin, PYY, or leptin play a direct role in the regulation of the hypothalamic-pituitary-ovarian axis, and if these signals can be altered by improving energy status secondary to increasing caloric intake and initiate the reversal of amenorrhea.

Since the passage of Title IX in the United States, opportunities for women to participate in physical activity (PA) and sport have dramatically increased. One of the earliest reports of menstrual irregularity in female athletes was published in 1962, and since then numerous studies have confirmed this finding in a wide range of athletes across a spectrum of various sports [1–4]. Since then, the prevalence of menstrual disturbances has been well described in both recreational runners and athletes [5, 6].

One of the earliest investigators to propose a mechanism to explain the high prevalence of menstrual disorders in athletes was Dr. Michelle Warren who suggested that 'energy drain' or the energetic cost of exercise may play a role in the onset of menstrual cycle perturbations in physically active women and athletes [7]. Since then, much has been published on the role of energy deficiency in the reapportioning of metabolic fuel away from reproduction and toward bodily functions such as cell maintenance, immune function and thermoregulation [8, 9]. This paper explores the etiology of menstrual disturbances in exercising women and the role of gut peptides and adipocytokines in this mechanism.

Menstrual Disturbances in Physically Active Women

Menstrual cycle perturbations are often observed in women who participate in PA ranging from recreational to competitive, and modest to strenuous exercise training [5, 6]. Exercise-related menstrual disturbances are manifested along a continuum of severity ranging from subtle disturbances like luteal phase defects (LPD) and anovulation in asymptomatic cycles of regular length, to increasingly severe menstrual disturbances like oligomenorrhea, and amenorrhea [6, 10, 11]. This continuum of menstrual disturbances is displayed in figure 1. Amenorrhea represents the most extreme presentation of menstrual irregularity and is described as 'functional hypothalamic amenorrhea' (FHA) when a disruption occurs at the level of the hypothalamus concomitant with exercise training [9, 12]. FHA is characterized by chronic hypoestrogenism and is associated with severe clinical sequelae such as stress fractures, low bone mineral density and a potential increase in the risk of premature cardiovascular disease [13–16]. Disordered eating, menstrual irregularities, and bone loss are interrelated medical conditions which comprise the syndrome known as the Female Athlete Triad [13]. Figure 2 displays the interrelatedness of disordered eating, reproductive suppression and compromised bone health associated with the Female Athlete Triad.

The severe menstrual disturbances observed in physically active women and athletes include amenorrhea and oligomenorrhea. Amenorrhea has been defined as the absence of menstruation and can be further subdivided into two categories: primary and secondary. Secondary amenorrhea occurs sometime after menarche and is conservatively defined as no menses for a minimum of 3 months [6, 9]. Amenorrhea in athletes is hypothalamic in origin, associated with reduced luteinizing hormone (LH) pulsatility, chronically suppressed ovarian steroids, and unaltered pituitary responsiveness to gonadotropin-releasing hormone (GnRH) in female athletes [12, 17]. Primary amenorrhea is defined as the absence of menstruation by 15 y in girls with secondary sex characteristics [18]. Oligomenorrhea is defined by irregular and inconsistent menstrual cycles of 36–90 days in length [6], and in athletes careful evaluation of the androgen environment should be considered to rule out irregular

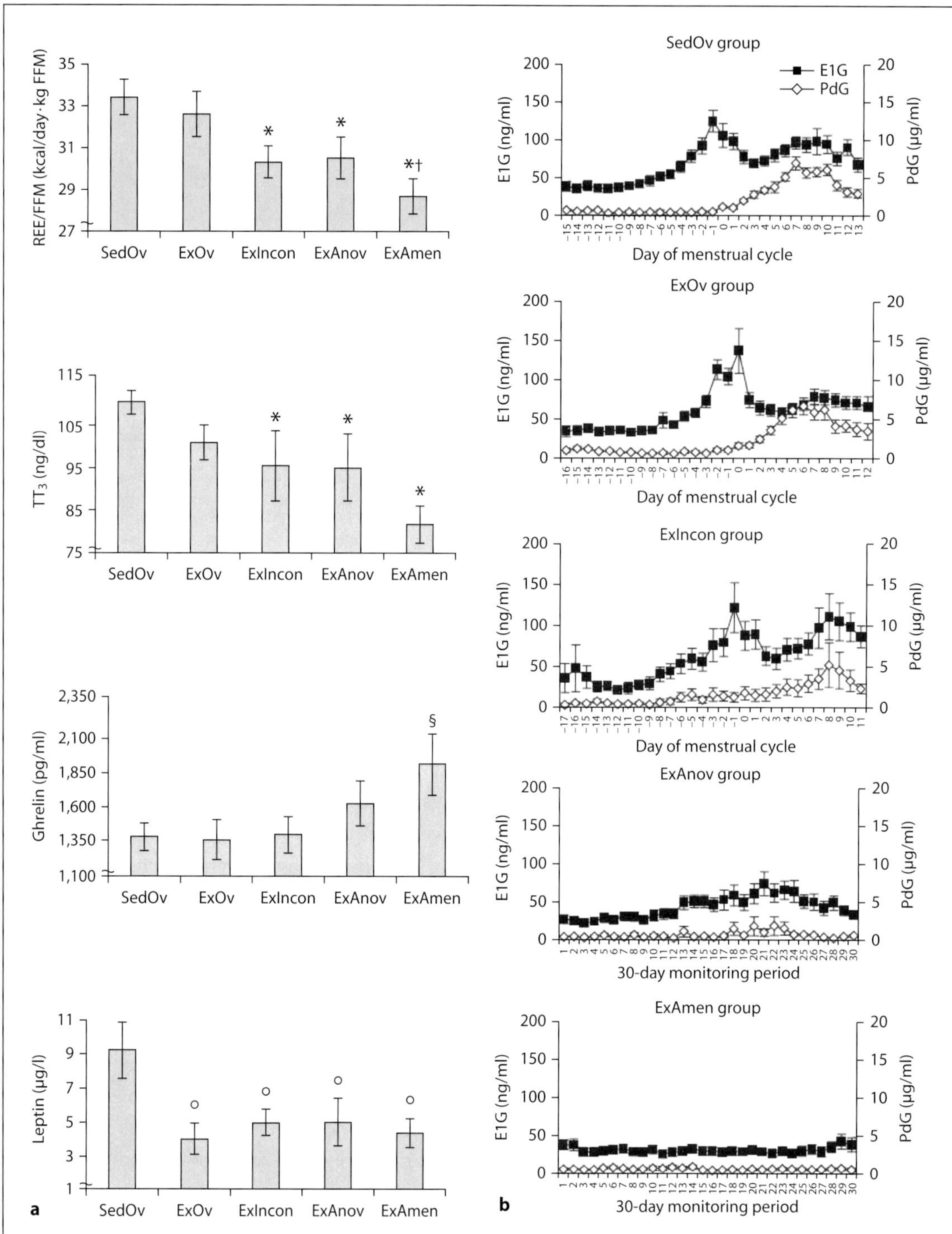
REE/FFM (kcal/day·kg FFM)
SedOv
ExOv
ExIncon
ExAnov
ExAmen
TT3 (ng/dl)
Ghrelin (pg/ml)
Leptin (µg/l)
a
SedOv group
ExOv group
ExIncon group
ExAnov group
ExAmen group
E1G
PdG
E1G (ng/ml)
PdG (µg/ml)
Day of menstrual cycle
30-day monitoring period
b

cycles associated with polycystic ovarian syndrome (PCOS) per se [19]. Since PCOS is the most common cause of infertility in women, it is not surprising that some athletes bring PCOS to the athletic environment where it fails to be diagnosed and since these women may present with oligomenorrhea or amenorrhea, they are perceived to be oligo-/amenorrheic secondary to an energy deficit, as opposed to PCOS [19].

Prevalence studies on amenorrhea in athletes have reported variable estimates ranging from 1 to 66% [1, 3, 4, 6, 20, 21]. Reported prevalence rates in females athletes are much greater than those observed in the general population of nonathletic, college-aged women [22, 23] largely attributable to the emphasis on the achievement of thin and lean physiques which may require low body weights and body fat percentages in sports such as figure skating, ballet, long-distance running and gymnastics. The prevalence of primary amenorrhea in a group of young triathletes was recently reported to be as high as 40% [24]. The prevalence of oligomenorrhea in athletes has reported to range from 9–40% [2, 3, 11, 25–28], which is higher than the prevalence rate observed in non-athletic women of 5–11% [23, 29].

The subtle menstrual disturbances observed in physically active women and athletes include anovulation and LPD. Anovulation is defined as the absence of an ovulatory event or LH peak in association with reduced estrogen levels and the absence of luteinization [5, 6, 30]. LPD is defined as short when the luteal phase length is less than 10 days [30], or inadequate when the sum of the 3-day mid-luteal peak pregnanediol glucoronide (PdG) is less than 10 μg/ml and when the PdG peak concentration is below 5 μg/ml [5, 6, 30, 31]. In women with LPD, there is inadequate luteinization to support implantation, since the latter is dependent on an adequate progestational effect [30]. Figure 1 displays the spectrum of menstrual disturbances observed in exercising women when described via daily hormone measures of urinary excretion of estrone-1 glucuronide (E1G) and PdG.

Fig. 1. **a** Metabolic changes of women with energy related menstrual cycle disturbances. Bar graph of REE per kilogram of fat-free mass (FFM) (kcal/day of REE per kg of FFM), triiodothyronine (TT_3, ng/dl), ghrelin (pg/ml), and leptin (μg/l) in the sedentary and exercising women grouped by menstrual status: sedentary with ovulatory cycles (SedOv), exercising with ovulatory cycles (ExOv), exercising with inconsistent cycles, i.e. some cycles with luteal phase defects or anovulatory cycles (ExIncon), exercising with consistent anovulatory cycles (ExAnov), and exercising with amenorrhea (ExAmen). $p < 0.05$, * ExAmen, ExAnov, ExIncon vs. SedOv; † ExAmen vs. ExOv; § ExAmen vs. SedOv, ExOv, ExIncon, ExAnov; and ° ExAmen, ExAnov, ExIncon, ExOv vs. SedOv. Results are expressed as mean ± SEM. **b** Composite graphs of menstrual status depicted by daily estrone 1-glucuronide (E1G, ng/ml) and pregnanediol glucuronide (PdG, μg/ml) concentrations in the sedentary and exercising women grouped by menstrual status. The E1G and PdG data for SedOv, ExOv, and ExIncon groups are aligned by the day of the LH peak, defined as day 0. The anovulatory (ExAnov) and amenorrheic (ExAmen) subjects' E1G and PdG data are aligned by chronological day of daily urinary hormone collections. The number of days depicted for the amenorrheic subjects is the mean cycle length of the menstruating subjects. Results are expressed as mean ± SEM. Reprinted from De Souza et al. [8], with permission.

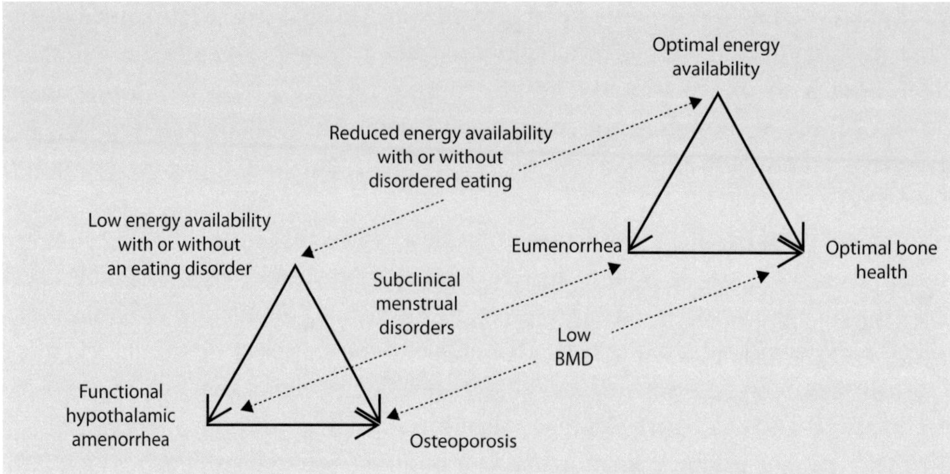

Fig. 2. The schematic displays the interrelatedness of disordered eating, reproductive suppression and compromised bone health associated with the Female Athlete Triad on a continuum from optimal (optimal energy availability, eumenorrhea, and optimal bone health) to most severe (low energy availability with or without an eating disorder, functional hypothalamic amenorrhea, and osteoporosis). Reprinted from Nattiv et al. [13], with permission.

LPD and anovulation represent the most common menstrual abnormality associated with exercise training and physical activity [5, 6]. The prevalence of LPD in athletes is much greater than that observed when compared to non-active or sedentary women. In a 3-month observational study, the prevalence of LPD and anovulation was found to be 48 and 79%, respectively, in recreationally active women [5]. More recently, we have confirmed these high prevalence rates [6]. Indeed, as many as 50% of 120 cycles evaluated in exercising women were abnormal (LPD or anovulation); whereas, only 4% of 48 cycles evaluated in sedentary women were abnormal [6]. The previous percentage is of concern because recreationally active women and athletes may be characterized by a menstrual disturbance without any clinical demonstration or symptoms of the abnormality since these disturbances occur in the face of normal cycle lengths. Because these abnormalities are inconspicuous, both clinicians and active women must be educated in order to understand and prevent these problems.

Etiology of Exercise-Related Menstrual Disturbances

Menstrual disturbances in physically active women have been casually linked to an energy deficiency where caloric intake is inadequate for exercise energy expenditure resulting in a suppressive effect on growth and reproduction [9]. The suppression of growth and reproductive function during conditions of a chronic energy deficiency is a well-recognized energy-conserving strategy intended to preserve fuel for more vital bodily processes, such as cellular maintenance, immune function and locomotion [9, 32]. Reproduction, in particular, is a physiologically costly process that requires significant energy reserves in order to sustain ovulatory function and adequate luteinization [33].

In exercising women, the evidence for a role of energy deficiency in the modulation of reproductive function has been generated from observational and cross-sectional studies of athletes and exercising women, and from prospective studies utilizing both short- and long-term designs. Evidence from observational and cross-sectional studies include data that demonstrate that exercising women with varying severity of menstrual disturbances are discriminated from each other based on their metabolic profile [8, 34, 35]. Indeed, we examined the evidence for alterations in resting energy expenditure (REE) and metabolic hormones in exercising women with menstrual disturbances ranging from subtle disturbances like LPD and anovulation to severe disturbances like amenorrhea [8]. We observed adaptations consistent with chronic energy deficiency, including reductions in REE and total triiodothyronine (TT_3) and elevations in ghrelin concentrations [8]. Moreover, these alterations were observed across the continuum of clinical menstrual disturbances in a dose-response manner consistent with the severity of the menstrual dysfunction observed. In a study of 49 premenopausal women, De Souza et al. [8] demonstrated that the above-mentioned energy deficiency increases in severity across the continuum of menstrual cycle disturbances such that the exercising women with amenorrhea, the most severe menstrual disturbance, had the lowest REE relative to fat free mass, the lowest TT_3 concentrations, and the highest ghrelin concentrations compared to the exercising women with subtle menstrual disturbances. The results of the study by De Souza et al. [8] are displayed in figure 1. Figure 3 summarizes the mild to severe perturbations in metabolic status across the range of menstrual perturbations observed in exercising women, highlighting the fact that metabolic alterations increase in severity as the menstrual perturbation becomes more severe.

Prospective studies of short-term 4- to 5-day manipulations of food intake and exercise energy expenditure in sedentary women have also been demonstrated to alter metabolic profiles and LH pulsatility in a dose-response fashion at varying levels of energy availability [36–38]. Prospective 2- to 3-month exercise training studies where energetic challenges were imposed in women [39, 40] by increasing energy expenditure and decreasing energy intake, demonstrated that these energetic challenges induced menstrual disturbances, including LPD, anovulation and delayed menses. Williams et al. [41, 42] also provided evidence for a causal relationship between energy availability and menstrual cyclicity by inducing amenorrhea in monkeys during exercise training and then by reversing the amenorrhea and restoring ovulation in the monkeys by increasing food intake without moderating the energy expenditure. The restoration of ovulation in the amenorrheic monkeys was related to the volumes

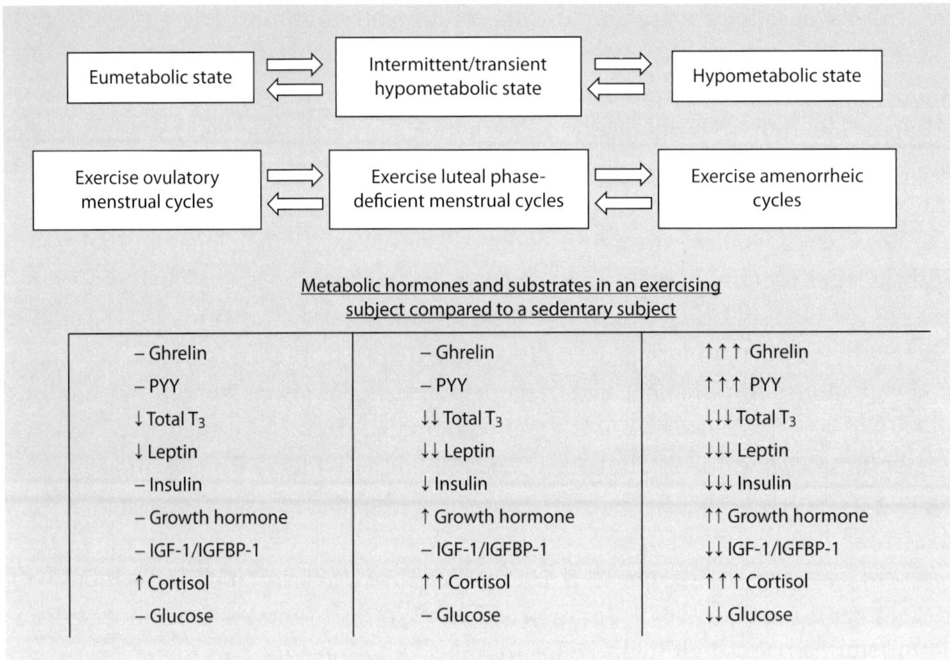

Fig. 3. The schematic displays the metabolic hormones and substrates that are altered in exercising women with ovulatory menstrual cycles, compared to exercising women with luteal phase-deficient menstrual cycles, and exercising women with amenorrhea. Reprinted from De Souza and Williams [9], with permission.

of calories consumed during refeeding such that the monkeys that ate the most calories resumed menses over the shortest interval [41]. Confirmation that the suppression of reproductive function was coupled to energy-conserving mechanisms was the observation that alterations in TT_3 was associated with both the induction and reversal of amenorrhea in the monkeys [41, 42].

Despite our understanding of the causal role of low energy availability in the induction of menstrual disturbances, appropriate practical guidelines of the optimal combination of dietary intake and exercise energy expenditure to maintain ovulation in exercising women remains undefined. Based on data in the experiments of Loucks et al. [38], it has been suggested that the threshold of energy available in physically active women must exceed 30 kcal/kg lean body mass/day to maintain normal LH pulsatility. More research is needed to confirm if this recommendation of energy availability translates to the maintenance of ovulatory function. Current efforts to review this issue and provide a set of guidelines for athletes and physically active women are underway by the Female Athlete Triad Coalition, an international consortium of professionals dedicated to optimizing the health of female athletes (www.femaleathletetriad.com).

Eating Behaviors, Gut Peptides, and Adipocytokines

In an effort to address a plausible mechanism for insufficient dietary intake in female athletes, much has been described regarding the physiological cues signaling food intake and psychological domains that control or modulate eating behavior. It is clear that in some cases where menstrual disturbances are secondary to an energy deficiency in athletic women, there is some form of disordered eating behavior that contributes to this condition [13, 43–45]. The disordered eating behavior in athletes often presents as a high drive for thinness or as the conscious restriction of caloric intake, often referred to as dietary cognitive restraint [43, 46].

Although significant relationships between disordered eating behaviors have been related to menstrual disturbances in female athletes, it should not be assumed that *every* athlete has a psychological profile consistent with such pathology. It is logical to question whether the physiological cues for hunger and satiety in exercising women are distorted and are not appropriately coordinated to detect and meet exercise energy needs, or if some other cognitive cues that drive food intake are altered. In an effort to examine some of these issues, the roles of gut peptides and adipocytokines, important signals of hunger and satiety in exercising women are reviewed.

Ghrelin

Ghrelin is a gastrointestinal hormone secreted by distinct endocrine cells of the stomach called X/A-like or ghrelin cells [47, 48]. Peripherally produced ghrelin can cross the blood-brain barrier and regulate the release of neuropeptide Y (NPY) and agouti-related protein (AgRP) from the arcuate nucleus in the hypothalamus [49]. Ghrelin activates the ghrelin receptors in the arcuate nucleus to upregulate the release of NPY and AgR as well suppress the activation of the pro-opiomelanocortin (POMC) and cocaine- and amphetamine-regulated transcript (CART) leading to an increase in hunger and food intake [49, 50]. Through these central mechanisms, ghrelin has been proposed to play a role in short-term energy homeostasis, and, interestingly, ghrelin is the only circulating peripheral orexigenic hormone known to stimulate appetite [50]. Ghrelin concentrations rise preprandially and fall postprandially in healthy individuals [51]. The rise in ghrelin concentrations before a meal is a physiological signal for hunger and the body's cue for meal initiation, and, interestingly, the rise in ghrelin concentrations and hunger occurs independent of food and time of day cues [52]. The rise in ghrelin concentrations across the day is related to previous meal caloric intake, meaning that if subsequent meal caloric intake is low then an elevated ghrelin profile, associated with the next meal, will occur [53]. Additionally, fasting ghrelin concentrations are demonstrated to be negatively correlated to 24-hour caloric intake [54]. Ghrelin concentrations decrease following caloric intake [53], and the decrease in ghrelin release is related to the amount of calories ingested [53]. Additionally, decreases in circulating ghrelin concentrations have been demonstrated to be related to carbohydrate intake [55] such that ghrelin concentrations decrease after consuming a carbohydrate rich meal, while protein and fat-rich meals result in an increase in circulating ghrelin concentrations. Ghrelin infusions during a buffet meal are associated with an increase in food intake [56]. Indeed, in 9 nonobese males and females, Wren et al. [56] intravenously infused ghrelin and demonstrated a 28% increase in caloric intake, indicating that the effects of circulating ghrelin concentrations are potent and can cause a large increase in appetite and food intake.

While ghrelin concentrations are tightly regulated by caloric intake, fasting circulating ghrelin concentrations are also negatively correlated to REE [54], indicating a role for ghrelin in regulating long-term energy homeostasis. Borer et al. [57] suggest that ghrelin concentrations respond rapidly to a negative energy balance, induced by either small meals or exercise. To this end, fasting ghrelin concentrations are elevated following weight loss due to diet and exercise in normal-weight premenopausal women [53].

While weight loss is an example of an energy deficiency, i.e. energy intake is less then energy expenditure in order to achieve weight loss, anorexia nervosa is an example of a more severe and chronic long-term energy deficiency. Anorexia nervosa is related to a cognitive suppression of food intake leading to a chronic energy deficiency. Ghrelin is chronically elevated in women with anorexia nervosa [58–61], supporting a role for ghrelin as a hormone involved in long-term energy homeostasis. Total ghrelin secretion over 12 h is elevated in women with anorexia nervosa compared to healthy controls and anorexic women fail to demonstrate a meal-induced reduction of ghrelin concentrations, indicating that ghrelin levels are chronically elevated in women with anorexia [58, 60]. Since ghrelin concentrations are consistently elevated in energy deficient models, ghrelin may prove to be an important marker of energy deficiency and chronic undernutrition.

Another population demonstrating an energy deficiency is exercising women with FHA. Since the etiology of exercise-associated FHA is based on an energy deficiency and energy conservation, women with exercise-associated FHA also display evidence for elevations in fasting ghrelin concentrations [8, 35] and as previously described, other evidence of metabolic suppression including a decrease in REE, and suppression of TT_3, insulin-like growth factor-1 and leptin concentrations and elevations in cortisol concentrations [8, 9]. Whether ghrelin concentrations are chronically elevated remains to be determined since no meal studies have been published to date in this population. Despite the finding that fasting ghrelin concentrations are elevated in exercising women with FHA [8, 35, 62–64], increased appetite and/or increased food intake has not been reported in these women. Additionally, Borer et al. [57] suggest that ghrelin concentrations respond rapidly to a negative energy balance induced by exercise, and while ghrelin concentrations parallel energy status, elevated ghrelin concentrations do not induce hunger, supporting the finding that exercising women with FHA do not have increased hunger despite their elevated fasting ghrelin concentration. Interestingly, a high drive for thinness has been reported in exercising women with FHA. Such women have elevated fasting ghrelin concentrations compared to women with a normal drive for thinness [65], indicating that if physiological hunger cues are elevated due to an energy deficiency, psychological cues, like a high drive for thinness, may act to suppress food intake.

Elevated ghrelin concentrations in exercising women with FHA and anorexia nervosa have been suggested to be related to a relative resistance to ghrelin [66]. Ghrelin administration stimulates appetite in healthy and obese individuals [67] and ghrelin has been suggested as a potential treatment for women with anorexia nervosa to pharmacologically increase food intake by modulating hunger and to assist with weight gain. However, Miljic et al. [68] administered ghrelin to women with anorexia and failed to observe an increase in hunger (measured by visual analog scales). The study [68] demonstrated that ghrelin administration may not be an effective treatment to increase food intake in women with anorexia nervosa and supports the premise that women with anorexia nervosa are resistant to the orexigenic effects of ghrelin. The results from Miljic et al. [68] would likely translate to women with FHA, i.e. exercising women with FHA are also likely resistant, at least to some extent, to the effects of elevated ghrelin. Ghrelin resistance may be a physiological phenomenon; however, it is likely that psychological components are also hindering the ability of ghrelin to simulate appetite. Similar to women with anorexia nervosa, the resistance to ghrelin in women with FHA may also be related to cognitive suppression of food intake observed in women with FHA with a high drive for thinness [65] and high dietary cognitive restraint [69].

Ghrelin and other metabolic and gastrointestinal hormones that are altered in women with amenorrhea may have a role in reproductive suppression [8, 35, 62]. Many investigations have explored the relationship between metabolic alterations and reproduction [32, 42, 70, 71]. Interestingly, metabolic and gastrointestinal hormones have the ability to cross the blood-brain barrier and interact with NPY/AgRP and POMC/CART in the arcuate nucleus to affect appetite and additionally, are also hypothesized to affect the hypothalamic-pituitary-ovarian axis [72]. A schematic of this hypothesis is shown in figure 4. Elevated ghrelin concentrations in women with FHA may be involved in reproductive suppression; a direct relationship between elevated ghrelin and reproductive suppression has been shown in multiple animal models [71, 73, 74]. Vulliemoz et al. [71] infused ghrelin in rhesus monkeys and demonstrated decreased LH pulse frequency, suggesting that GnRH activity is downregulated by elevated circulating ghrelin concentrations. Messini et al. [75] investigated the effect of a single ghrelin injection in normally menstruating women and failed to demonstrate any effect of the acute ghrelin injection on LH, while other investigators [76, 77] have demonstrated that LH secretion is suppressed in men following a longer ghrelin administration. While many hormones are altered in women with FHA, ghrelin may be a hormone that, while attempting to regulate long-term energy homeostasis, contributes to the down regulation of GnRH, i.e. elevated ghrelin may contribute to the etiology of FHA.

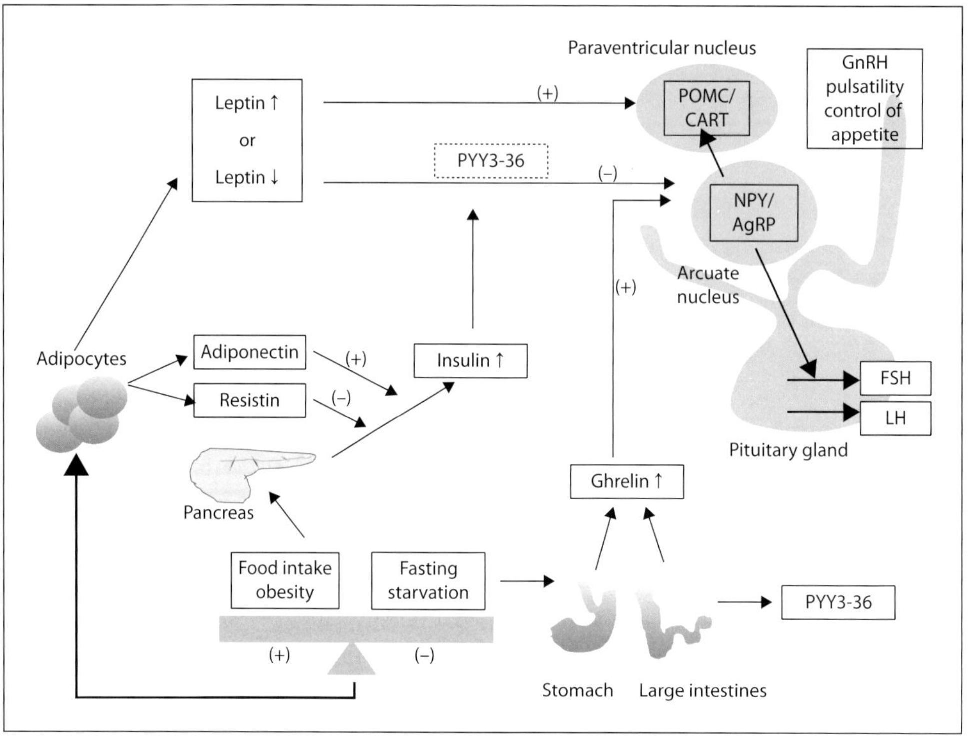

Fig. 4. Metabolic and gastrointestinal hormones including leptin, insulin, ghrelin and peptide YY (PYY_{3-36}) that all have the ability to cross the blood-brain barrier and interact with neuropeptide Y (NPY) and agouti-related protein (AgRP) and pro-opiomelanocortin (POMC) and cocaine- and amphetamine regulated transcript (CART) in the arcuate nucleus to affect appetite and, additionally, are also hypothesized to affect the hypothalamic-pituitary-ovarian axis impacting follicle stimulating hormone (FSH) and luteinizing hormones (LH). Reprinted from Budak et al. [72], with permission.

Peptide YY

Peptide YY (PYY) is a gastrointestinal peptide secreted from the endocrine L cells of the intestine in response to caloric intake [78–81]. Similar to ghrelin, PYY can cross the blood brain barrier and act centrally at the level of the arcuate nucleus to contribute to eating behavior. While ghrelin stimulates the releases of NPY and AgRP to increase hunger and food intake, PYY_{3-36} (the active form of PYY) activates the Y2 receptors to inhibit NPY and AgRP, as well as activate POMC and CART, to decrease hunger and food intake [78, 82]. Through these central mechanisms, PYY has a role in short-term energy homeostasis, and unique from ghrelin, causes a decrease in appetite. PYY concentrations rise in response to a caloric load after a meal [79, 81, 83] and stay elevated for several hours [80]. Peak PYY concentrations are achieved in proportion to the amount of calories ingested [79, 84]. While caloric intake is followed by an elevation in PYY concentration, two to three days of fasting suppresses PYY

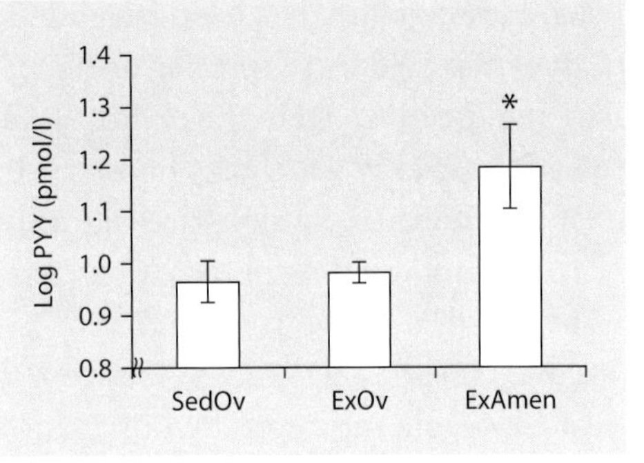

Fig. 5. Fasting total peptide YY (PYY) concentrations in women who are sedentary and have ovulatory menstrual cycles (SedOv) and exercising women who have ovulatory menstrual cycles (ExOv), compared to exercising women with amenorrhea (ExAmen). * $p < 0.05$, ExAmen vs. SedOv and ExOv. Results are expressed as mean ± SEM. Reprinted from Scheid et al. [62], with permission.

concentrations by 40–60% below baseline in lean men and women [85]. PYY infusion during a buffet meal is associated with a decrease in food intake [82]. Batterham et al. [82] infused PYY_{3-36} in 12 healthy nonobese men and women and demonstrated that caloric intake was decreased by 30%, indicating that the effects of PYY include large reductions in appetite and food intake.

Fasting PYY concentrations are tightly regulated by caloric intake and negatively correlated with BMI [86], suggesting a role for PYY in regulating long-term energy homeostasis. While the weight loss literature is inconsistent and difficult to interpret, obese children who lose weight have an increase in circulating PYY concentrations [87], and obese adults who lose weight have reported decreased PYY concentrations [88, 89]. However, women with anorexia nervosa, a population exhibiting a reduction in body weight and energy deficiency, have consistently been observed to exhibit elevated fasting PYY concentrations [66, 88, 90]. Similar to women with anorexia nervosa, exercising women with FHA secondary to an energy deficiency also demonstrate elevated fasting PYY concentrations [62, 91]. These data support the premise that specific energy deficient populations, including women with anorexia nervosa and exercising women with FHA, have elevated fasting PYY concentrations, and PYY likely plays a role in regulating long-term energy homeostasis in these energy deficient models.

Interestingly, while fasting ghrelin, an orexigenic peptide, is elevated in women with FHA, PYY, an anorexigenic peptide, is paradoxically also elevated in women with anorexia nervosa and exercising women with FHA. Scheid et al. [62] reported that fasting concentrations of PYY are elevated in exercising women with FHA compared to both exercising women with ovulatory cycles and sedentary women with ovulatory cycles. Figure 5 summarizes the findings from Scheid and colleagues. Many other investigators have also demonstrated that fasting PYY concentrations are elevated in anorexic women [66, 88, 90]. Elevated PYY concentrations are presumably related to an energy deficiency, as demonstrated by the negative correlations of PYY with BMI [86] and REE [62]. The interpretation of these findings likely suggest that PYY could simply be a biomarker of long-term energy homeostasis related to energy deficiency, particularly in women with anorexia nervosa and exercising women with

FHA. Elevated PYY has been suggested to facilitate decreased food intake secondary to the anorexigenic properties of PYY. Misra et al. [66] have suggested that elevated PYY may be involved in the pathogenesis of anorexia nervosa and this may also play a role in the energy deficiency observed in exercising women with FHA [62]. However, if PYY is indeed a physiological signal that is suppressing food intake, this signal may be compounding disordered eating behaviors in these women.

In addition to the role of ghrelin in regulating the hypothalamic-pituitary-ovarian axis, there is evidence to suggest that elevated PYY concentrations play a role in downregulating reproduction in women with anorexia nervosa and exercising women with FHA. Similar to ghrelin, PYY has the ability to cross the blood-brain barrier and interact with NPY/AgRP and POMC/CART in the arcuate nucleus and can modulate appetite and food intake, and via these same mechanisms, is hypothesized to affect the hypothalamic-pituitary-ovarian axis [72] (fig. 4). Women with anorexia nervosa and FHA both experience suppressed reproductive function and elevated PYY concentrations [62, 66, 91]. There is also evidence that PYY may be directly participating in the downregulation of reproductive function; however, to date, the evidence for this direct relationship has only been shown in animal models [92, 93]. Investigations in Syrian hamsters have shown that infusions of PYY inhibit estrous [92]. While Fernandez-Fernandez et al. [93] administered PYY_{3-36} to rats and observed a decrease in LH release, future research is needed to investigate if findings in these rodent models translate to human models, and if elevated circulating PYY concentrations in women with anorexia and exercising women with FHA are contributing to the downregulation of GnRH and LH pulsatility.

Lastly, elevated PYY concentrations may play a role in the uncoupled relationship between elevated ghrelin and food intake in energy deficient women. Exercising women with FHA demonstrate elevated ghrelin concentrations [8, 35, 62–64] and experience a relative ghrelin resistance, i.e. women with FHA express behaviors including restricting food intake even in the presence of elevated physiological signals, like ghrelin, to increase food intake. As previously noted, PYY is elevated in exercising women with FHA and in women with anorexia nervosa [62, 91] and PYY has been shown to inhibit ghrelin neurons [94]. As pointed out by Misra et al. [66], elevated PYY in the presence of elevated ghrelin may also cause a relative ghrelin resistance in these women. A comprehensive gastrointestinal profile in energy deficient women will be important to investigate to determine if there are physiological signals to explain the psychological behavior of suppressed food intake in energy-deficient women.

Leptin

Leptin is an adipocytokine that has been identified as a peripheral signal of energy status and is an important long-term regulator of food intake [95]. Similar to ghrelin and PYY, leptin can cross the blood-brain barrier and act on the arcuate nucleus in the hypothalamus [96]. Leptin activates the leptin receptors to inhibit NPY and AgRP, as well activate POMC/CART to decrease food intake [96]. Through these central mechanisms, ghrelin, leptin and PYY all participate in regulating energy homeostasis. Both animal [97, 98] and human [99] models have shown that a leptin deficiency can cause severe alterations in energy homeostasis leading to obesity, indicating that leptin is necessary for the long-term regulation of body weight. Leptin resistance is proposed to perpetuate obesity [100], i.e. a leptin resistance leads to a decrease in satiety, and an increase in food intake and weight gain and could play a role in obesity. Weight loss due to dieting decreases circulating leptin concentrations [101], indicating that a loss in fat mass is associated with a decrease in leptin secretion from adipose tissue. Although leptin is correlated with body fat stores and weight loss [101, 102], days of fasting suppresses fasting leptin concentrations independent of declines in fat mass [103]. As such, leptin also acts as a short-term regulator of energy homeostasis since food intake stimulates leptin production while fasting inhibits leptin production [104].

Leptin is involved in the long-term regulation of energy homeostasis and is tightly correlated with body fat. Women with anorexia nervosa exhibiting chronic energy deficiency, have consistently been observed to exhibit suppressed fasting leptin concentrations [105]. Audi et al. [106] cross-sectionally evaluated three groups of women with anorexia nervosa – (1) underweight and amenorrheic, (2) weight-recovered and amenorrheic, and (3) weight-recovered and eumenorrheic – and demonstrated that leptin concentrations were suppressed in the women who were underweight, indicating that increasing body weight and leptin concentrations alone are not sufficient to reverse amenorrhea, but are likely important factors for the resumption of menses. To this end, Kopp et al. [107] demonstrated that a critical leptin concentration or threshold was necessary for regular menses to occur in underweight women. Indeed, since leptin receptors have been identified at all levels of the hypothalamic-pituitary-ovarian axis, and since there is in vivo and in vitro confirmation of an effect of leptin on the axis, strong support for a role of leptin in reproductive function is supported [108, 109].

Similar to women with anorexia nervosa, women with FHA also demonstrate suppressed leptin concentrations [110, 111]. Miller et al. [110] demonstrated that women with FHA have suppressed leptin concentrations compared to age-, weight-, and body fat-matched eumenorrheic controls and that suppressed leptin concentrations may be related to low levels of caloric intake and/or suppressed fat intake in women with FHA compared to the controls. Similarly, ballet dancers demonstrate a higher incidence of amenorrhea and have suppressed leptin concentrations compared to age-, weight-, and body fat-matched controls [112].

Studies investigating the relationship between leptin and amenorrhea are difficult to interpret because, although leptin may have a role in regulating reproduction [70], leptin concentrations are tightly regulated by body fat stores [101]. Suppressed leptin

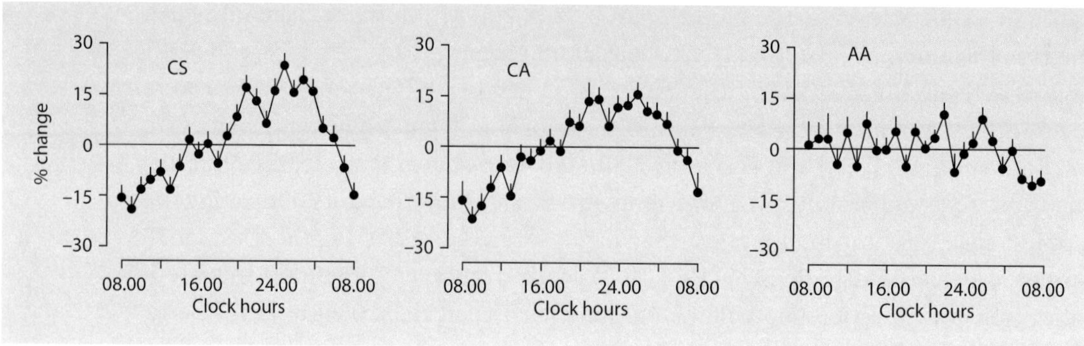

Fig. 6. Leptin changes during a 24-hour period as percentage changes from the 24-hour mean leptin concentration in three groups: sedentary women with eumenorrhea (CS), exercising women with eumenorrhea (CA), and exercising women with amenorrhea (AA). Results are expressed as mean ± SEM. Reprinted from Laughlin and Yen [111], with permission.

concentrations in women with amenorrhea are often reflective of decreased body fat [64, 113]. For example, when an exercising control group is used to evaluate leptin concentrations in women with FHA, leptin concentrations are suppressed in both exercising women with FHA and exercising control women compared to sedentary women [35, 114]. De Souza et al. [8, 35] demonstrated that women with exercise-associated FHA have suppressed leptin concentrations similar to the suppressed leptin concentrations observed in ovulatory exercising women, i.e. leptin concentrations are more tightly associated with body fat than menstrual status [8, 35]. Interestingly, Laughlin and Yen [111] demonstrate that exercising women with FHA have similar fasting leptin concentrations to athletic controls, but that exercising women with FHA have an absent 24-hour diurnal pattern of leptin, while the athletic controls have a normal diurnal pattern of 24-hour leptin concentrations (fig. 6), indicating that measuring fasting leptin concentrations may not be sensitive enough to discriminate circulating leptin concentrations in lean populations.

While there is indirect evidence in animal and human models to suggest that ghrelin and PYY both participate in regulating reproduction, researchers have provided ample evidence to suggest that leptin is involved in regulating the hypothalamic-pituitary-ovarian axis in humans [70, 106, 107] (fig. 4). While it is likely that many factors modulate reproduction and signal adequate energy status to the arcuate nucleus, a critical leptin environment is likely a key signal for reproductive function in humans [107]. Welt et al. [70] administered recombinant human leptin to 8 women with FHA and demonstrated an increase in mean LH pulse frequency. Additionally, the leptin administration caused an increase in follicular growth, including an increase in the number of dominant follicles which was associated with an ovulatory menstrual cycle in three of the eight participants during the three month intervention. Welt et al. [70], for the first time in humans, demonstrated that leptin is a key signal for reproductive function and that leptin is one of the metabolic hormones and indicators of energy homeostasis that regulates the hypothalamic-pituitary-ovarian axis. While the findings of Welt and colleagues indicate that leptin is an important regulator of reproductive function, the findings also, potentially, have therapeutic implications [70]. However, caution should be exercised because while three months of recombinant leptin treatment clearly improved reproductive function in some women with FHA, leptin therapy also caused a decrease in body weight and fat mass in a population who are already typically underweight [70]. Increased caloric intake in women with FHA may be a more appropriate method of improving energy status, body weight, body fat and potentially leptin levels to subsequently have an improvement in reproductive status. Increased caloric intake in exercising women with FHA has been demonstrated to reverse amenorrhea [115, 116]; however, to date, no studies in humans have investigated what specific metabolic signals upregulate reproduction and reverse amenorrhea in exercising women with FHA during a period of increased caloric intake. Future studies are needed to investigate the role of ghrelin, PYY, and leptin in regulating the hypothalamic-pituitary-ovarian axis, and determine if these signals can be altered by improving energy status via increased caloric intake.

Conclusions

Exercising women with FHA display adaptations consistent with chronic energy deficiency, including alterations in gut peptides and adipocytokines. Ghrelin, PYY, and leptin all have the ability to cross the blood-brain barrier and, in the hypothalamus, can modulate appetite and food intake, and are hypothesized to affect the hypothalamic-pituitary-ovarian axis. Elevated ghrelin and PYY concentrations and suppressed leptin concentrations therefore appear to be involved in the etiology of FHA. Future studies are needed to determine if ghrelin, PYY, or leptin are playing a direct role in regulating the hypothalamic-pituitary-ovarian axis, and if these signals can be altered by improving energy status secondary to increasing caloric intake and initiate the reversal of amenorrhea.

References

1 Baker ER, Mathur RS, Kirk RF, Williamson HO: Female runners and secondary amenorrhea: correlation with age, parity, mileage, and plasma hormonal and sex-hormone-binding globulin concentrations. Fertil Steril 1981;36:183–187.

2 Beals KA, Manore MM: Disorders of the female athlete triad among collegiate athletes. Int J Sport Nutr Exerc Metab 2002;12:281–293.

3 Dale E, Gerlach DH, Wilhite AL: Menstrual dysfunction in distance runners. Obstet Gynecol 1979;54:47–53.

4 Feicht CB, Johnson TS, Martin BJ, Sparkes KE, Wagner WW Jr: Secondary amenorrhoea in athletes. Lancet 1978;ii:1145–1146.

5 De Souza MJ, Miller BE, Loucks AB, Luciano AA, Pescatello LS, Campbell CG, Lasley BL: High frequency of luteal phase deficiency and anovulation in recreational women runners: blunted elevation in follicle-stimulating hormone observed during luteal-follicular transition. J Clin Endocrinol Metab 1998;83:4220–4232.
6 De Souza MJ, Toombs RJ, Scheid JL, O'Donnell E, West SL, Williams NI: High prevalence of subtle and severe menstrual disturbances in exercising women: confirmation using daily hormone measures. Hum Reprod 2010;25:491–503.
7 Warren MP: The effects of exercise on pubertal progression and reproductive function in girls: J Clin Endocrinol Metab 1980;51:1150–1157.
8 De Souza MJ, Lee DK, VanHeest JL, Scheid JL, West SL, Williams NI: Severity of energy-related menstrual disturbances increases in proportion to indices of energy conservation in exercising women. Fertil Steril 2007;88:971–975.
9 De Souza MJ, Williams NI: Physiological aspects and clinical sequelae of energy deficiency and hypoestrogenism in exercising women. Hum Reprod Update 2004;10:433–448.
10 Beitins IZ, McArthur JW, Turnbull BA, Skrinar GS, Bullen BA: Exercise induces two types of human luteal dysfunction: confirmation by urinary free progesterone. J Clin Endocrinol Metab 1991;72: 1350–1358.
11 Brooks-Gunn J, Warren MP, Hamilton LH: The relation of eating problems and amenorrhea in ballet dancers. Med Sci Sports Exerc 1987;19:41–44.
12 Williams NI: Lessons from experimental disruptions of the menstrual cycle in humans and monkeys. Med Sci Sports Exerc 2003;35:1564.
13 Nattiv A, Loucks AB, Manore MM, Sanborn CF, Sundgot-Borgen J, Warren MP: American College of Sports Medicine position stand: the female athlete triad. Med Sci Sports Exerc 2007;39:1867–1882.
14 O'Donnell E, Harvey PJ, De Souza MJ: Relationships between vascular resistance and energy deficiency, nutritional status and oxidative stress in oestrogen deficient physically active women. Clin Endocrinol 2009;70:294–302.
15 O'Donnell E, Harvey PJ, Goodman JM, De Souza MJ: Long-term estrogen deficiency lowers regional blood flow, resting systolic blood pressure, and heart rate in exercising premenopausal women. Am J Physiol Endocrinol Metab 2007;292: E1401–E1409.
16 Zeni Hoch A, Dempsey RL, Carrera GF, et al: Is there an association between athletic amenorrhea and endothelial cell dysfunction? Med Sci Sports Exerc 2003;35:377–383.
17 Veldhuis JD, Evans WS, Demers LM, Thorner MO, Wakat D, Rogol AD: Altered neuroendocrine regulation of gonadotropin secretion in women distance runners. J Clin Endocrinol Metab 1985;61:557–563.
18 ASRM: Current evaluation of amenorrhea: the Practice Committee of the American Society of Reproductive Medicine. Fertil Steril 2006;86: S148–S155.
19 Awdishu S, Williams NI, Laredo SE, De Souza MJ: Oligomenorrhoea in exercising women: a polycystic ovarian syndrome phenotype or distinct entity? Sports Med 2009;39:1055–1069.
20 Sanborn CF, Martin BJ, Wagner WW Jr: Is athletic amenorrhea specific to runners? Am J Obstet Gynecol 1982;143:859–861.
21 Schwartz B, Cumming DC, Riordan E, Selye M, Yen SS, Rebar RW: Exercise-associated amenorrhea: a distinct entity? Am J Obstet Gynecol 1981;141:662–670.
22 Pettersson F, Fries H, Nillius SJ: Epidemiology of secondary amenorrhea. I. Incidence and prevalence rates. Am J Obstet Gynecol 1973;117:80–86.
23 Singh KB: Menstrual disorders in college students. Am J Obstet Gynecol 1981;140:299–302.
24 Hoch AZ, Stavrakos JE, Schimke JE: Prevalence of female athlete triad characteristics in a club triathlon team. Arch Phys Med Rehabil 2007;88:681–682.
25 Shangold MM, Levine HS: The effect of marathon training upon menstrual function. Am J Obstet Gynecol 1982;143:862–869.
26 Glass AR, Deuster PA, Kyle SB, Yahiro JA, Vigersky RA, Schoomaker EB: Amenorrhea in Olympic marathon runners. Fertil Steril 1987;48:740–745.
27 Cobb KL, Bachrach LK, Greendale G, et al: Disordered eating, menstrual irregularity, and bone mineral density in female runners. Med Sci Sports Exerc 2003;35:711–719.
28 Nichols JF, Rauh MJ, Barrack MT, Barkai HS, Pernick Y: Disordered eating and menstrual irregularity in high school athletes in lean-build and non-lean-build sports. Int J Sport Nutr Exerc Metab 2007;17:364–377.
29 Bachmann GA, Kemmann E: Prevalence of oligomenorrhea and amenorrhea in a college population. Am J Obstet Gynecol 1982;144:98–102.
30 Jordan J, Craig K, Clifton DK, Soules MR: Luteal phase defect: the sensitivity and specificity of diagnostic methods in common clinical use. Fertil Steril 1994;62:54–62.
31 Santoro N, Crawford SL, Allsworth JE, et al: Assessing menstrual cycles with urinary hormone assays. Am J Physiol Endocrinol Metab 2003; 284: E521–E530.
32 Wade GN, Schneider JE, Li HY: Control of fertility by metabolic cues. Am J Physiol 1996;270:E1.

33 Wade GN, Schneider JE: Metabolic fuels and reproduction in female mammals. Neurosci Biobehav Rev 1992;16:235.
34 De Souza MJ: Menstrual disturbances in athletes: a focus on luteal phase defects. Med Sci Sports Exerc 2003;35:1553.
35 De Souza MJ, Leidy HJ, O'Donnell E, Lasley B, Williams NI: Fasting ghrelin levels in physically active women: relationship with menstrual disturbances and metabolic hormones. J Clin Endocrinol Metab 2004;89:3536–3542.
36 Williams NI, Young JC, McArthur JW, Bullen B, Skrinar GS, Turnbull B: Strenuous exercise with caloric restriction: effect on luteinizing hormone secretion. Med Sci Sports Exerc 1995;27:1390.
37 Loucks AB: The response of luteinizing hormone pulsatility to 5 days of low energy availability disappears by 14 years of gynecological age. J Clin Endocrinol Metab 2006;91:3158–3164.
38 Loucks AB, Thuma JR: Luteinizing hormone pulsatility is disrupted at a threshold of energy availability in regularly menstruating women. J Clin Endocrinol Metab 2003;88:297–311.
39 Bullen BA, Skrinar GS, Beitins IZ, von Mering G, Turnbull BA, McArthur JW: Induction of menstrual disorders by strenuous exercise in untrained women. N Engl J Med 1985;312:1349–1353.
40 Williams NI, Bullen BA, McArthur JW, Skrinar GS, Turnbull BA: Effects of short-term strenuous endurance exercise upon corpus luteum function. Med Sci Sports Exerc 1999;31:949–958.
41 Williams NI, Caston-Balderrama AL, Helmreich DL, Parfitt DB, Nosbisch C, Cameron JL: Longitudinal changes in reproductive hormones and menstrual cyclicity in cynomolgus monkeys during strenuous exercise training: abrupt transition to exercise-induced amenorrhea. Endocrinology 2001; 142:2381.
42 Williams NI, Helmreich DL, Parfitt DB, Caston-Balderrama A, Cameron JL: Evidence for a causal role of low energy availability in the induction of menstrual cycle disturbances during strenuous exercise training. J Clin Endocrinol Metab 2001;86:5184.
43 Beals KA, Hill AK: The prevalence of disordered eating, menstrual dysfunction, and low bone mineral density among US collegiate athletes. Int J Sport Nutr Exerc Metab 2006;16:1–23.
44 Sundgot-Borgen J: Risk and trigger factors for the development of eating disorders in female elite athletes. Med Sci Sports Exerc 1994;26:414–419.
45 Sanborn CF, Horea M, Siemers BJ, Dieringer KI: Disordered eating and the female athlete triad. Clin Sports Med 2000;19:199–213.
46 Sundgot-Borgen J: Weight and eating disorders in elite athletes: Scand J Med Sci Sports 2002;12:259–260.
47 Kojima M, Hosoda H, Date Y, Nakazato M, Matsuo H, Kangawa K: Ghrelin is a growth-hormone-releasing acylated peptide from stomach. Nature 1999;402:656–660.
48 Date Y, Kojima M, Hosoda H, et al: Ghrelin, a novel growth hormone-releasing acylated peptide, is synthesized in a distinct endocrine cell type in the gastrointestinal tracts of rats and humans. Endocrinology 2000;141:4255.
49 Kamegai J, Tamura H, Shimizu T, Ishii S, Sugihara H, Wakabayashi I: Chronic central infusion of ghrelin increases hypothalamic neuropeptide Y and Agouti-related protein mRNA levels and body weight in rats. Diabetes 2001;50:2438–2443.
50 Wren AM, Bloom SR: Gut hormones and appetite control. Gastroenterology 2007;132:2116–2130.
51 Cummings DE, Purnell JQ, Frayo RS, Schmidova K, Wisse BE, Weigle DS: A preprandial rise in plasma ghrelin levels suggests a role in meal initiation in humans. Diabetes 2001;50:1714–1719.
52 Cummings DE, Frayo RS, Marmonier C, Aubert R, Chapelot D: Plasma ghrelin levels and hunger scores in humans initiating meals voluntarily without time- and food-related cues. Am J Physiol Endocrinol Metab 2004;287:E297–E304.
53 Leidy HJ, Williams NI: Meal energy content is related to features of meal-related ghrelin profiles across a typical day of eating in non-obese premenopausal women. Horm Metab Res 2006;38:317.
54 St-Pierre DH, Faraj M, Karelis AD, et al: Lifestyle behaviours and components of energy balance as independent predictors of ghrelin and adiponectin in young non-obese women. Diabetes Matab 2006; 32:131.
55 Erdmann J, Topsch R, Lippl F, Gussmann P, Schusdziarra V: Postprandial response of plasma ghrelin levels to various test meals in relation to food intake, plasma insulin, and glucose. J Clin Endocrinol Metab 2004;89:3048–3054.
56 Wren AM, Seal LJ, Cohen MA, et al: Ghrelin enhances appetite and increases food intake in humans. J Clin Endocrinol Metab 2001;86:5992.
57 Borer KT, Wuorinen E, Ku K, Burant C: Appetite responds to changes in meal content, whereas ghrelin, leptin, and insulin track changes in energy availability. J Clin Endocrinol Metab 2009;94:2290–2298.
58 Nedvidkova J, Krykorkova I, Bartak V, Papezova H, Gold PW, Alesci S, Pacak K: Loss of meal-induced decrease in plasma ghrelin levels in patients with anorexia nervosa. J Clin Endocrinol Metab 2003;88: 1678.

59 Tolle V, Kadem M, Bluet-Pajot MT, et al: Balance in ghrelin and leptin plasma levels in anorexia nervosa patients and constitutionally thin women. J Clin Endocrinol Metab 2003;88:109.
60 Misra M, Miller KK, Herzog DB, et al: Growth hormone and ghrelin responses to an oral glucose load in adolescent girls with anorexia nervosa and controls. J Clin Endocrinol Metab 2004;89:1605.
61 Misra M, Miller KK, Stewart V, Hunter E, Kuo K, Herzog DB, Klibanski A: Ghrelin and bone metabolism in adolescent girls with anorexia nervosa and healthy adolescents. J Clin Endocrinol Metab 2005; 90:5082.
62 Scheid JL, Williams NI, West SL, VanHeest JL, De Souza MJ: Elevated PYY is associated with energy deficiency and indices of subclinical disordered eating in exercising women with hypothalamic amenorrhea. Appetite 2009;52:184–192.
63 Schneider LF, Warren MP: Functional hypothalamic amenorrhea is associated with elevated ghrelin and disordered eating. Fertil Steril 2006;86:1744–1749.
64 Christo K, Cord J, Mendes N, Miller KK, Goldstein MA, Klibanski A, Misra M: Acylated ghrelin and leptin in adolescent athletes with amenorrhea, eumenorrheic athletes and controls: a cross-sectional study. Clin Endocrinol 2008;69:628–633.
65 De Souza MJ, Hontscharuk R, Olmsted M, Kerr G, Williams NI: Drive for thinness score is a proxy indicator of energy deficiency in exercising women. Appetite 2007;48:359–367.
66 Misra M, Miller KK, Tsai P, et al: Elevated peptide YY levels in adolescent girls with anorexia nervosa. J Clin Endocrinol Metab 2006;91:1027–1033.
67 Druce MR, Wren AM, Park AJ, et al: Ghrelin increases food intake in obese as well as lean subjects. Int J Obes 2005;29:1130.
68 Miljic D, Pekic S, Djurovic M, et al: Ghrelin has partial or no effect on appetite, growth hormone, prolactin, and cortisol release in patients with anorexia nervosa. J Clin Endocrinol Metab 2006;91:1491–1495.
69 Vescovi JD, Scheid JL, Hontscharuk R, De Souza MJ: Cognitive dietary restraint: impact on bone, menstrual and metabolic status in young women. Physiol Behav 2008;95:48–55.
70 Welt CK, Chan JL, Bullen J, et al: Recombinant human leptin in women with hypothalamic amenorrhea. N Engl J Med 2004;351:987.
71 Vulliemoz NR, Xiao E, Xia-Zhang L, Germond M, Rivier J, Ferin M: Decrease in luteinizing hormone pulse frequency during a five-hour peripheral ghrelin infusion in the ovariectomized rhesus monkey. J Clin Endocrinol Metab 2004;89:5718–5723.
72 Budak E, Fernandez Sanchez M, Bellver J, Cervero A, Simon C, Pellicer A: Interactions of the hormones leptin, ghrelin, adiponectin, resistin, and PYY3–36 with the reproductive system. Fertil Steril 2006;85:1563.
73 Fernandez-Fernandez R, Tena-Sempere M, Navarro VM, Barreiro ML, Castellano JM, Aguilar E, Pinilla L: Effects of ghrelin upon gonadotropin-releasing hormone and gonadotropin secretion in adult female rats: in vivo and in vitro studies. Neuroendocrinology 2005;82:245–255.
74 Furuta M, Funabashi T, Kimura F: Intracerebroventricular administration of ghrelin rapidly suppresses pulsatile luteinizing hormone secretion in ovariectomized rats. Biochem Biophys Res Commun 2001;288:780.
75 Messini CI, Dafopoulos K, Chalvatzas N, Georgoulias P, Messinis IE: Effect of ghrelin on gonadotrophin secretion in women during the menstrual cycle. Hum Reprod 2009;24:976–981.
76 Kluge M, Schussler P, Uhr M, Yassouridis A, Steiger A: Ghrelin suppresses secretion of luteinizing hormone in humans. J Clin Endocrinol Metab 2007;92: 3202–3205.
77 Lanfranco F, Bonelli L, Baldi M, Me E, Broglio F, Ghigo E: Acylated ghrelin inhibits spontaneous luteinizing hormone pulsatility and responsiveness to naloxone but not that to gonadotropin-releasing hormone in young men: evidence for a central inhibitory action of ghrelin on the gonadal axis. J Clin Endocrinol Metab 2008;93:3633–3639.
78 Batterham RL, Cohen MA, Ellis SM, et al: Inhibition of food intake in obese subjects by peptide YY3–36. N Engl J Med 2003;349:941–948.
79 Huda MS, Wilding JP, Pinkney JH: Gut peptides and the regulation of appetite. ObesRev 2006;7:163–182.
80 Adrian TE, Ferri GL, Bacarese-Hamilton AJ, Fuessl HS, Polak JM, Bloom SR: Human distribution and release of a putative new gut hormone, peptide YY. Gastroenterology 1985;89:1070–1077.
81 Kim BJ, Carlson OD, Jang HJ, Elahi D, Berry C, Egan JM: Peptide YY is secreted after oral glucose administration in a gender-specific manner. J Clin Endocrinol Metab 2005;90:6665–6671.
82 Batterham RL, Cowley MA, Small CJ, et al: Gut hormone PYY(3–36) physiologically inhibits food intake. Nature 2002;418:650.
83 Korner J, Bessler M, Cirilo LJ, Conwell IM, Daud A, Restuccia NL, Wardlaw SL: Effects of Roux-en-Y gastric bypass surgery on fasting and postprandial concentrations of plasma ghrelin, peptide YY, and insulin. J Clin Endocrinol Metab 2005;90:359–365.

84 Degen L, Oesch S, Casanova M, Graf S, Ketterer S, Drewe J, Beglinger C: Effect of peptide YY3–36 on food intake in humans. Gastroenterology 2005;129: 1430.

85 Chan JL, Stoyneva V, Kelesidis T, Raciti P, Mantzoros CS: Peptide YY levels are decreased by fasting and elevated following caloric intake but are not regulated by leptin. Diabetologia 2006;49:169.

86 Guo Y, Ma L, Enriori PJ, et al: Physiological evidence for the involvement of peptide YY in the regulation of energy homeostasis in humans. Obesity 2006;14:1562–1570.

87 Roth CL, Enriori PJ, Harz K, Woelfle J, Cowley MA, Reinehr T: Peptide YY is a regulator of energy homeostasis in obese children before and after weight loss. J Clin Endocrinol Metab 2005;90:6386–6391.

88 Pfluger PT, Kampe J, Castaneda TR, et al: Effect of human body weight changes on circulating levels of peptide YY and peptide YY3–36. J Clin Endocrinol Metab 2007;92:583–588.

89 Lien LF, Haqq AM, Arlotto M, et al: The STEDMAN project: biophysical, biochemical and metabolic effects of a behavioral weight loss intervention during weight loss, maintenance, and regain. OMICS 2009;13:21–35.

90 Nakahara T, Kojima S, Tanaka M, et al: Incomplete restoration of the secretion of ghrelin and PYY compared to insulin after food ingestion following weight gain in anorexia nervosa. J Psychiatr Res 2007;41:814–820.

91 Russell M, Stark J, Nayak S, Miller KK, Herzog DB, Klibanski A, Misra M: Peptide YY in adolescent athletes with amenorrhea, eumenorrheic athletes and non-athletic controls. Bone 2009;45:104–109.

92 Keene AC, Jones JE, Wade GN, Corp ES: Forebrain sites of NPY action on estrous behavior in Syrian hamsters. Physiol Behav 2003;78:711–716.

93 Fernandez-Fernandez R, Aguilar E, Tena-Sempere M, Pinilla L: Effects of polypeptide YY(3–36) upon luteinizing hormone-releasing hormone and gonadotropin secretion in prepubertal rats: in vivo and in vitro studies. Endocrinology 2005;146:1403–1410.

94 Riediger T, Bothe C, Becskei C, Lutz TA: Peptide YY directly inhibits ghrelin-activated neurons of the arcuate nucleus and reverses fasting-induced c-Fos expression. Neuroendocrinology 2004;79:317–326.

95 Keim NL, Stern JS, Havel PJ: Relation between circulating leptin concentrations and appetite during a prolonged, moderate energy deficit in women. Am J Clin Nutr 1998;68:794–801.

96 Schwartz MW, Morton GJ: Obesity: keeping hunger at bay. Nature 2002;418:595.

97 Zhang Y, Proenca R, Maffei M, Barone M, Leopold L, Friedman JM: Positional cloning of the mouse obese gene and its human homologue. Nature 1994; 372:425–432.

98 Pelleymounter MA, Cullen MJ, Baker MB, Hecht R, Winters D, Boone T, Collins F: Effects of the obese gene product on body weight regulation in ob/ob mice. Science 1995;269:540–543.

99 Montague CT, Farooqi IS, Whitehead JP, et al: Congenital leptin deficiency is associated with severe early-onset obesity in humans. Nature 1997;387: 903–908.

100 Scarpace PJ, Zhang Y: Leptin resistance: a predisposing factor for diet-induced obesity. Am J Physiol Regul Integr Comp Physiol 2009;296:R493–R500.

101 Maffei M, Halaas J, Ravussin E, et al: Leptin levels in human and rodent: measurement of plasma leptin and ob RNA in obese and weight-reduced subjects. Nat Med 1995;1:1155–1161.

102 Weigle DS, Duell PB, Connor WE, Steiner RA, Soules MR, Kuijper JL: Effect of fasting, refeeding, and dietary fat restriction on plasma leptin levels. J Clin Endocrinol Metab 1997;82:561–565.

103 Chan JL, Heist K, DePaoli AM, Veldhuis JD, Mantzoros CS: The role of falling leptin levels in the neuroendocrine and metabolic adaptation to short-term starvation in healthy men. J Clin Invest 2003; 111:1409–1421.

104 Budak E, Fernandez Sanchez M, Bellver J, Cervero A, Simon C, Pellicer A: Interactions of the hormones leptin, ghrelin, adiponectin, resistin, and PYY3–36 with the reproductive system. Fertil Steril 2006;85:1563–1581.

105 Grinspoon S, Gulick T, Askari H, et al: Serum leptin levels in women with anorexia nervosa. J Clin Endocrinol Metab 1996;81:3861–3863.

106 Audi L, Mantzoros CS, Vidal-Puig A, Vargas D, Gussinye M, Carrascosa A: Leptin in relation to resumption of menses in women with anorexia nervosa. Mol Psychiatry 1998;3:544–547.

107 Kopp W, Blum WF, von Prittwitz S, et al: Low leptin levels predict amenorrhea in underweight and eating disordered females. Mol Psychiatry 1997;2:335–340.

108 Yu WH, Kimura M, Walczewska A, Karanth S, McCann SM: Role of leptin in hypothalamic-pituitary function. Proc Natl Acad Sci USA 1997;94: 1023–1028.

109 Sone M, Osamura RY: Leptin and the pituitary. Pituitary 2001;4:15–23.

110 Miller KK, Parulekar MS, Schoenfeld E, Anderson E, Hubbard J, Klibanski A, Grinspoon SK: Decreased leptin levels in normal weight women with hypothalamic amenorrhea: the effects of body composition and nutritional intake. J Clin Endocrinol Metab 1998;83:2309–2312.

111 Laughlin GA, Yen SS: Hypoleptinemia in women athletes: absence of a diurnal rhythm with amenorrhea. J Clin Endocrinol Metab 1997;82:318–321.
112 Kaufman BA, Warren MP, Dominguez JE, Wang J, Heymsfield SB, Pierson RN: Bone density and amenorrhea in ballet dancers are related to a decreased resting metabolic rate and lower leptin levels. J Clin Endocrinol Metab 2002;87:2777–2783.
113 Warren MP, Voussoughian F, Geer EB, Hyle EP, Adberg CL, Ramos RH: Functional hypothalamic amenorrhea: hypoleptinemia and disordered eating. J Clin Endocrinol Metab 1999;84:873–877.
114 Schneider LF, Monaco SE, Warren MP: Elevated ghrelin level in women of normal weight with amenorrhea is related to disordered eating. Fertil Steril 2008;90:121–128.
115 Dueck CA, Matt KS, Manore MM, Skinner JS: Treatment of athletic amenorrhea with a diet and training intervention program. International J Sport Nutr 1996;6:24.
116 Kopp-Woodroffe SA, Manore MM, Dueck CA, Skinner JS, Matt KS: Energy and nutrient status of amenorrheic athletes participating in a diet and exercise training intervention program. Int J Sport Nutr 1999;9:70–88.

Mary Jane De Souza, PhD, FACSM
Women's Health and Exercise Laboratory
Noll Laboratory, Department of Kinesiology, Penn State University
University Park, PA 16802 (USA)
Tel. +1 814 863 0045, Fax +1 814 865 4602, E-Mail mjd34@psu.edu

Jürimäe J, Hills AP, Jürimäe T (eds): Cytokines, Growth Mediators and Physical Activity in Children during Puberty.
Med Sport Sci. Basel, Karger, 2010, vol 55, pp 103–113

Influence of Ghrelin and Adipocytokines on Bone Mineral Density in Adolescent Female Athletes with Amenorrhea and Eumenorrheic Athletes

Melissa Russell · Madhusmita Misra

Pediatric Endocrine and Neuroendocrine Units, Massachusetts General Hospital, Boston, Mass., USA

Abstract

Adolescent female athletes are at increased risk for low bone mineral density (BMD) secondary to exercise-induced hypogonadism. Of particular concern is that the adolescent years are also a critical time for bone accrual, and deficits incurred during this period could lead to suboptimal peak bone mass acquisition and subsequent fracture risk in later life. Although weight-bearing exercise is typically associated with an increase in BMD, amenorrheic athletes have lower BMD than eumenorrheic athletes and nonathletic controls as a consequence of low energy availability and subsequent hypogonadism. It is important to recognize that critical interactions exist between net energy availability and the hypothalamo-pituitary-gonadal (H-P-G) axis that are key to the development of a hypogonadal state when energy intake cannot keep pace with expenditure. While the link between energy availability and gonadtotropin pulsatility patterns is well established, the actual metabolic signals that link the two are less clear. Decreased energy availability in athletes is associated with decreases in fat mass, and alterations in adipokines (such as leptin and adiponectin) and fat-regulated hormones (such as ghrelin and peptide YY). These hormones impact the H-P-G axis in animal models, and it is possible that in athletes alterations in fat-related hormones signal the state of energy availability to the hypothalamus and contribute to suppression of gonadotropin pulsatility, hypothalamic amenorrhea and consequent decreased BMD. A better understanding of pathways linking low energy availability with functional hypothalamic amenorrhea and low BMD is critical for the development of future therapeutic strategies addressing these issues in amenorrheic athletes.

The adolescent years are characterized by marked increases in bone mass accrual in association with rising levels of growth hormone (GH), insulin-like growth factor-1 (IGF-1) and gonadal steroids. Of importance, more than 90% of peak bone mass is

Supported in part by NIH grant R01HD060827.

achieved by 18 years of age, and peak bone mass is an important determinant of bone health and fracture risk in later life [1]. A lower than expected rate of bone accrual leads to not only low bone mineral density (BMD) Z-scores, but also suboptimal peak bone mass and possibly increased fracture risk in later years.

Conditions associated with decreased rates of bone mass accrual in adolescence include those characterized by decreased secretion of hormones such as GH, IGF-1 and gonadal steroids, and increased secretion of hormones such as cortisol and thyroxine. In addition, alterations in certain adipokines, such as leptin and adiponectin, and peptides that are impacted by changes in BMI and fat mass, such as ghrelin, peptide YY (PYY) and insulin, can impact bone metabolism. Physical exercise is a positive determinant of bone mass accrual in healthy adolescents. However, excessive exercise, particularly in the setting of associated hypogonadism, leads to low BMD in adolescents as well as in adults. Marked alterations in adipokines and fat-regulated hormones have been described in amenorrheic athletes [2, 3], and these alterations and their impact on the hypothalamo-pituitary-gonadal (H-P-G) axis and on bone metabolism are described below.

Bone Metabolism in Adolescent Amenorrheic and Eumenorrheic Athletes and Nonathletic Controls

Many studies have reported that adult amenorrheic athletes have lower bone density than normally menstruating athletes [4–7], and in adolescents, endurance activities such as running have been associated with an increased risk of fractures [8]. There are limited data, however, regarding bone metabolism in adolescent athletes.

Within adolescent endurance athletes, we have shown that amenorrheic athletes have significantly lower bone density compared with eumenorrheic athletes and also nonathletic controls [9]. In a study of 21 amenorrheic adolescent athletes, 18 eumenorrheic athletes, and 18 controls, we demonstrated that amenorrheic athletes had lower bone density Z-scores at the spine and whole body compared with eumenorrheic athletes and nonathletic controls [9]. The amenorrheic athletes also had lower hip bone density Z-scores compared with eumenorrheic athletes. In addition, Z-scores for height adjusted measures of bone density, such as spine bone mineral apparent density (BMAD) and whole body bone mineral content for height (WB BMC/Ht) were lower in amenorrheic athletes compared with eumenorrheic athletes and controls. Lower spine bone density in amenorrheic athletes was a consequence of lower BMC for bone area indicative of lighter bones, whereas, lower WB bone density was a consequence of lower bone area for height, indicative of thinner bones. Importantly, levels of bone formation and bone resorption markers were lower in amenorrheic athletes compared with controls, suggestive of a reduced bone turnover state. This is in contrast to normal adolescence, which is a state of increased bone turnover (at least in early adolescence).

The two groups of athletes in the study did not differ for activity level, suggesting that factors other than intensity and duration of exercise determine which athletes will develop amenorrhea. The amenorrheic athletes did have lower body mass index (BMI) and fat mass than the eumenorrheic athletes, and the prevalence of disordered eating was much higher in the amenorrheic (62%) compared with the eumenorrheic group (11%). These data suggest that decreased energy availability from decreased caloric intake may contribute to lower BMI and fat mass and subsequent functional hypothalamic amenorrhea in amenorrheic athletes. In a regression model that included the diagnostic category, IGF-1 levels, activity level, bone age, BMI and lean mass, most of these covariates (except activity level) were independent determinants of bone density measures. These data emphasize the impact of the hypogonadal state and overall state of nutrition on bone metabolism in female adolescent athletes.

Similarly, in adult athletes, amenorrhea has been associated with lower bone density [4–7], and lower energy availability (as evidenced by higher scores for disordered eating) has been determined to be an important predictor of lower bone density measures [4]. Importantly, not all forms of excessive activity are associated with low bone density even when there is associated amenorrhea. For example, amenorrheic gymnasts do not have lower bone density than non-exercising controls [10, 11]. This has been postulated to be a consequence of differences in the nature of exercise. Gymnastics is a non-repetitive impact loading sport, as opposed to running, which is associated with repetitive impact and an endurance sport. The latter is less likely to manifest beneficial effects of mechanical loading on bone, and is more likely to be associated with low bone density, particularly when associated with low energy availability and hypogonadism.

Recent studies in anorexia nervosa, a state of severe negative energy balance, have shown that low bone mass accrual during the adolescent years can be followed by increases in bone mass after recovery of weight and menses [12]. However, catch-up is not complete, and this further raises concerns of a suboptimal peak bone mass despite subsequent attainment of a positive state of energy balance in adolescent athletes. Given this incomplete catch-up, therapeutic strategies may be necessary to optimize bone mass accrual, even while recovery from the low energy availability state is being optimized. In order to develop the appropriate therapeutic strategies, it is critical to develop a better understanding of the pathophysiology underlying low bone density in conditions of reduced energy availability, and of factors that contribute to hypogonadism, as well as other determinants of low bone density.

Factors Contributing to Low Bone Density in Amenorrheic Adolescent Athletes

The early adolescent years are characterized by increased bone turnover as a consequence of rising levels of GH and IGF-1, both of which are bone anabolic hormones [13,

14] and cause endocortical bone formation. Subsequently, rising levels of estrogen have anti-resorptive effects and reduce endosteal bone resorption. These pubertal changes are responsible for bone modeling and the bone mass accrual that is so characteristic of puberty. Low IGF-1 levels in athletes who are in a state of markedly reduced energy availability and the associated hypogonadism could cause marked decreases in rates of bone accrual, leading to low bone mineral density. Of concern, as many as 23.5% of adolescent athletes are at risk for amenorrhea [15]. In our studies, we have noted that low IGF-1 levels and hypogonadism are important determinants of low bone density in athletes [9]. Similarly, other studies in adults have indicated that hypogonadism in athletes is associated with decreased bone density and increased fracture risk [4, 16–19].

There are a lot of data to indicate that patterns of gonadotropin pulsatility change when energy availability falls below a critical threshold of 30 kcal/kg lean body mass/day [20]. Recent endeavors have aimed at examining metabolic signals that link low energy availability and impaired gonadotropin secretion, and fat mass and fat-related hormones are possible candidates. In our study, amenorrheic athletes had significantly lower fat mass than eumenorrheic athletes [2, 3]. We have also previously shown that increases in fat mass predict recovery of the H-P-G axis in girls with anorexia nervosa, a more severe state of energy deficit [21]. Therefore, it is likely that hormones that are secreted by fat or regulated by fat have an impact on the H-P-G axis. Interestingly, many hormones that are secreted or regulated by fat also have an impact on bone metabolism in in vitro and animal studies. Adipokines, such as leptin [22–25] and adiponectin [26–29], and hormones that are altered when body fat changes, such as ghrelin [30, 31] and PYY [32–34], can impact both the H-P-G axis and bone metabolism, and may be important links between net energy availability, reproductive status and bone mineral density.

Adipokines in Female Athletes

Decreased energy availability can result from increased energy expenditure, decreased energy intake or both [20], and is associated with low fat mass and a suppression of the H-P-G axis. This leads to low levels of gonadal steroids and a decreased rate of bone mass accrual. Associated with low fat mass are low levels of the adipokine, leptin [35–37], and high levels of another adipokine, adiponectin [38, 39]; hormones that likely signal information about available energy stores to the hypothalamus.

Leptin is primarily produced in adipocytes and its circulating levels are highly correlated with body fat content [35]. Levels decrease with weight loss and increase as BMI and body fat increase [36, 37, 40]. Sufficient fat mass is thought to be necessary for normal reproductive function, although the threshold of fat mass necessary for normal menses may differ from individual to individual. Leptin-deficient animals and humans who fail to undergo pubertal development have pubertal onset once leptin is administered [41]. This suggests that leptin facilitates GnRH stimulated

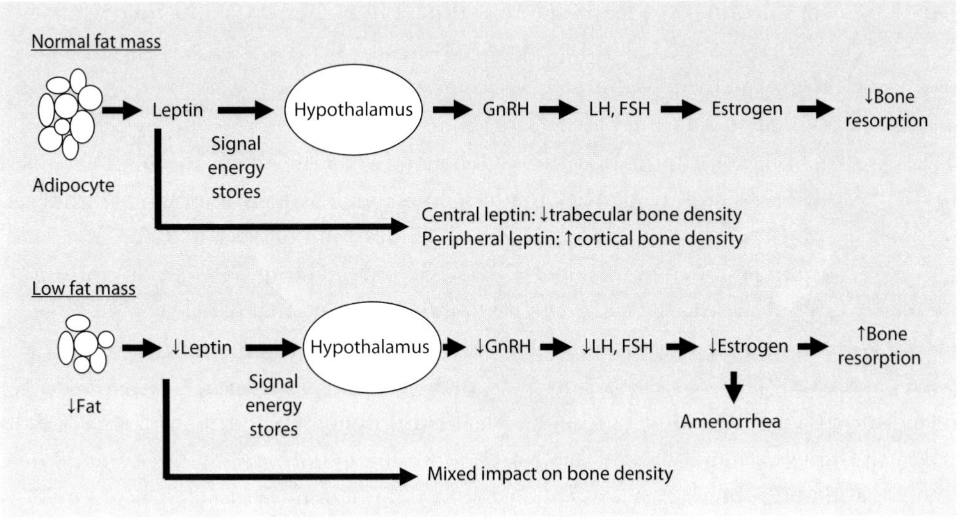

Fig. 1. Proposed impact of leptin on gonadotropin secretion and bone in conditions of normal versus low fat mass.

gonadotropin and gonadal steroid production, and that low leptin levels, as seen in athletes, could lead to hypogonadism and associated bone mineral density deficits. We have shown that leptin levels are significantly lower in adolescent amenorrheic athletes when compared with eumenorrheic athletes and controls [2], and low leptin levels are a positive predictor of levels of gonadal steroids, particularly estradiol, even after controlling for potential confounders. These data are also consistent with a study by Welt et al. [22] in which the authors demonstrated a resumption of ovulatory cycles following recombinant human leptin administration in 3 of 8 women with hypothalamic amenorrhea despite an overall reduction in body weight.

While low leptin levels in amenorrheic athletes can impact bone density through induction of a hypogonadal state, a direct role of leptin on bone cannot be ruled out. Leptin-deficient ob/ob mice have a decrease in trabecular bone mass when leptin is administered intracerebroventricularly [23], an effect mediated by beta-2-adrenergic activation. However, there appears to be a dichotomy in the effect of leptin on bone depending on whether it is administered centrally or peripherally. Contrary to central effects, peripherally administered leptin causes an increase in cortical bone mass [24, 25]. In addition, central leptin may also positively impact cortical bone by inducing GH secretion. In humans, studies examining associations of leptin and bone have shown variable results. Overall, leptin deficiency has been associated with increased [23], decreased [25], or site variable [24] bone mass. Figure 1 shows a speculated pathway of leptin induced effects on gonadal steroids and bone mineral density.

Adiponectin is the most abundant product secreted from adipocytes. In contrast to leptin, adiponectin levels are low in obesity [38] and variable in low weight conditions

[42, 43]. Adiponectin gene expression within adipocytes typically increases with weight loss and is associated with improved insulin sensitivity [39]. In vitro studies have demonstrated that adiponectin suppresses gonadotropin secretion [29] and activates both osteoblasts and osteoclasts [27, 28]. A common progenitor cell in bone marrow gives rise to adipocytes and osteoblasts [44, 45]. When adiponectin binds to the AdipoR1 receptor, mesenchymal progenitor cells within the marrow undergo osteoblast proliferation and differentiation, while adipogenesis is inhibited [28]. However, adiponectin can also increase RANKL and decrease OPG levels causing an increase in osteoclastic activity [27]. In adult men and women, as well as in postmenopausal women and adolescents with anorexia nervosa, high adiponectin levels have been associated with low bone density [42, 46, 47], suggesting that bone resorptive effects may trump bone formation effects. We did not find significant differences in adiponectin levels in adolescent amenorrheic athletes compared with eumenorrheic athletes and non-athletic controls [3]. However, adiponectin was a significant predictor of levels of testosterone. Contrary to our expectations and in vitro studies [29], the association between adiponectin and testosterone was positive (and not negative). We found no association between adiponectin and bone density measures in our athletes and non-athletic controls.

Hormones that May Be Regulated by Body Fat Content

Appetite-regulating hormones such as ghrelin and PYY are predicted inversely by BMI and fat mass. Ghrelin, one of the first orexigenic hormones to be discovered [48, 49], is secreted primarily by the P/D1 cells in the fundus of the stomach. Levels rise during periods of fasting and are low following food intake and in obesity, suggesting that ghrelin may signal the state of energy availability. Ghrelin levels rise in adults following exercise [50, 51] and are also high in anorexia nervosa [52, 53]. We evaluated ghrelin levels in amenorrheic adolescent athletes, eumenorrheic athletes, and nonathletic controls, and found that amenorrheic athletes had significantly higher ghrelin levels than eumenorrheic athletes and controls even after controlling for BMI [2]. In addition, we found an inverse relationship between levels of ghrelin and gonadal steroids leading us to postulate that ghrelin levels may differentiate between athletes who will or will not develop functional hypothalamic amenorrhea. These data are also consistent with studies in animals and humans that demonstrate a suppression of gonadotropin pulsatility following ghrelin administration [31, 54]. Figure 2 demonstrates the effect of food intake on ghrelin levels.

Ghrelin binds to and activates the neuropeptide Y (NPY) and agouti-related peptide-producing neurons in the arcuate nucleus of the hypothalamus, and therefore stimulates appetite and food intake [48, 55]. It is also a GH secretagogue [56, 57], and GH promotes bone formation. Therefore, ghrelin may have an effect on bone mass accrual by stimulating GH secretion. In addition, osteoblasts express

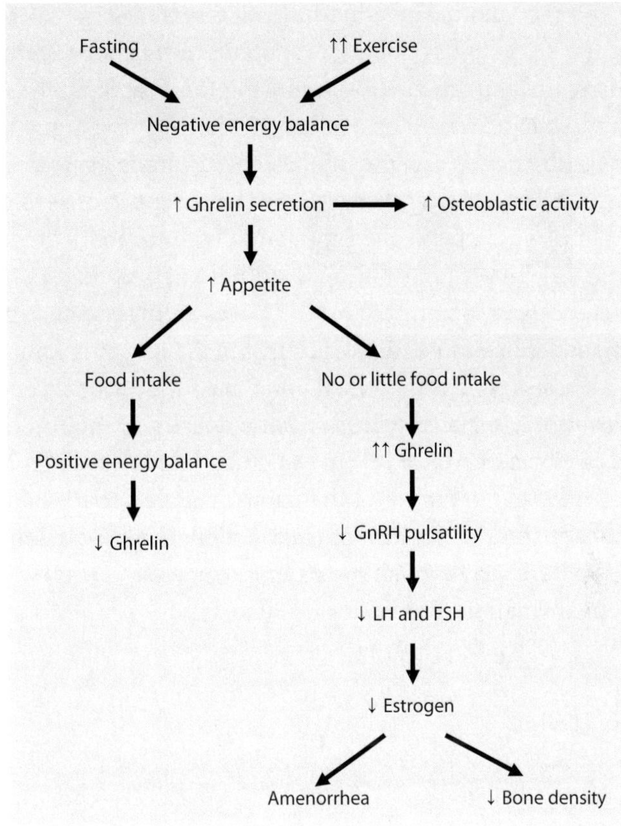

Fig. 2. Effect of energy balance and ghrelin on gonadotropin secretion and bone.

the ghrelin receptor (GHS-R1a), and ghrelin can stimulate osteoblast proliferation and differentiation [30]. Therefore, ghrelin may affect bone mass accrual through mechanisms independent of the GH-IGF-1 axis. In a study of adolescent girls with anorexia nervosa and controls, we previously reported that serum ghrelin levels predicted bone mineral density independent of body composition, the GH-IGF-1 axis, and estradiol in healthy adolescent girls but not in girls with anorexia nervosa [58]. Thus, ghrelin appears to be involved in pathways that are both detrimental and beneficial to the process of bone mass accrual. While high ghrelin levels may contribute to the hypogonadal state and subsequently to low bone density, ghrelin may stimulate osteoblastic activity through GH-dependent or GH-independent mechanisms. The overall impact of these processes is still not clearly understood. In our study of adolescent amenorrheic and eumenorrheic athletes, ghrelin was not an independent predictor of bone density measures, but did emerge as an independent and negative predictor of markers of bone formation and bone resorption, suggesting that high ghrelin levels may contribute to the low bone turnover state in amenorrheic athletes [3].

PYY is another peptide hormone secreted by gut neuroendocrine cells involved in the signaling of energy availability. It is anorexigenic and secreted by the L cells of the distal intestine [59] following food intake [60], and promotes satiety by binding to the Y2 receptor of NPY in the hypothalamus and inhibiting NPY secretion [61]. PYY levels are low in obesity [62] and elevated in low energy availability states such as anorexia nervosa [34]. We have reported elevated levels of PYY in adolescent athletes with amenorrhea compared with eumenorrheic athletes and nonathletic controls [3]. Importantly, animal studies suggest that PYY may suppress gonadotropin secretion, and in our cohort, PYY was an inverse and independent predictor of levels of gonadal steroids. Importantly, the Y2 receptor knockout mouse, which would be PYY resistant, has increased bone mass [32]. Consistent with this model, PYY excess has been associated with low bone density in models of low energy availability such as anorexia nervosa [34]. In our study of adolescent athletes, PYY was a negative and independent predictor of the bone formation marker PINP and of lumbar bone mineral apparent density Z-scores [3]. Thus, high PYY levels in adolescent athletes may contribute to low bone density by suppressing the H-P-G axis and also by reducing bone formation.

Conclusion

Adolescent female athletes are at increased risk for incurring bone mineral density deficits at a critical period of bone mass accrual. Interactions between energy balance, reproductive function and bone mass accrual are interlinked and complex. Hormones produced by adipocytes and gut neuroendocrine cells are important signals of energy balance and play a major role in the control of the H-P-G axis and bone metabolism. Current research to better understand the complex pathways involved in these processes is promising, and with improved understanding of the metabolic and hormonal links between energy availability, reproduction and bone, new therapeutic options should become possible to treat the hypogonadism and low bone density characteristic of amenorrheic athletes.

References

1 Bachrach L: Acquisition of optimal bone mass in childhood and adolescence. Trends Endocrinol Metab 2001;12:22–28.

2 Christo K, Cord J, Mendes N, et al: Acylated ghrelin and leptin in adolescent athletes with amenorrhea, eumenorrheic athletes and controls: a cross-sectional study. Clin Endocrinol (Oxf) 2008;69:628–633.

3 Russell M, Stark J, Nayak S, et al: Peptide YY in adolescent athletes with amenorrhea, eumenorrheic athletes and non-athletic controls. Bone 2009;45: 104–109.

4 Cobb K, Bachrach L, Greendale G, et al: Disordered eating, menstrual irregularity, and bone mineral density in female runners. Med Sci Sports Exerc 2003;35:711–719.

5 Myburgh H, Hutchins J, Fataar A, Hough S, Noakes T: Low bone mineral density is an etiologic factor for stress fractures in athletes. Ann Intern Med 1990;113:754–759.
6 Myburgh K, Bachrach L, Lewis B, Kent K, Marcus R: Low bone mineral density at axial and appendicular sites in amenorrheic athletes. Med Sci Sports Exerc 1993;25:1197–1202.
7 Pettersson U, Stalnacke B, Ahlenius G, Henriksson-Larsen K, Lorentzon R: Low bone mass density at multiple skeletal sites, including the appendicular skeleton in amenorrheic runners. Calcif Tissue Int 1999;64:117–125.
8 Loud KJ, Gordon CM, Micheli LJ, Field AE: Correlates of stress fractures among preadolescent and adolescent girls. Pediatrics 2005;115:e399–e406.
9 Christo K, Prabhakaran R, Lamparello B, et al: Bone metabolism in adolescent athletes with amenorrhea, athletes with eumenorrhea, and control subjects. Pediatrics 2008;121:1127–1136.
10 Robinson TL, Snow-Harter C, Taaffe DR, et al: Gymnasts exhibit higher bone mass than runners despite similar prevalence of amenorrhea and oligomenorrhea. J Bone Miner Res 1995;10:26–35.
11 Snow C, Rosen C, Robinson T: Serum IGF-I is higher in gymnasts than runners and predicts bone and lean mass. Med Sci Sports Exerc 2000;32:1902–1907.
12 Misra M, Prabhakaran R, Miller KK, et al: Weight gain and restoration of menses as predictors of bone mineral density change in adolescent girls with anorexia nervosa-1. J Clin Endocrinol Metab 2008;93:1231–1237.
13 Ohlsson C, Bengtsson BA, Isaksson OG, Andreassen TT, Slootweg MC: Growth hormone and bone. Endocr Rev 1998;19:55–79.
14 Rauch F: Bone accrual in children: adding substance to surfaces. Pediatrics 2007;119(suppl 2):S137–S140.
15 Nichols JF, Rauh MJ, Lawson MJ, Ji M, Barkai HS: Prevalence of the female athlete triad syndrome among high school athletes. Arch Pediatr Adolesc Med 2006;160:137–142.
16 Drinkwater BL, Bruemner B, Chesnut CH 3rd: Menstrual history as a determinant of current bone density in young athletes. JAMA 1990;263:545–548.
17 Jones KP, Ravnikar VA, Tulchinsky D, Schiff I: Comparison of bone density in amenorrheic women due to athletics, weight loss, and premature menopause. Obstet Gynecol 1985;66:5–8.
18 Rencken ML, Chesnut CH 3rd, Drinkwater BL: Bone density at multiple skeletal sites in amenorrheic athletes. JAMA 1996;276:238–240.
19 Wolman RL, Clark P, McNally E, Harries M, Reeve J: Menstrual state and exercise as determinants of spinal trabecular bone density in female athletes. BMJ 1990;301:516–518.
20 Loucks AB, Verdun M, Heath EM: Low energy availability, not stress of exercise, alters LH pulsatility in exercising women. J Appl Physiol 1998;84:37–46.
21 Misra M, Prabhakaran R, Miller KK, et al: Role of cortisol in menstrual recovery in adolescent girls with anorexia nervosa. Pediatr Res 2006;59:598–603.
22 Welt CK, Chan JL, Bullen J, et al: Recombinant human leptin in women with hypothalamic amenorrhea. N Engl J Med 2004;351:987–997.
23 Ducy P, Amling M, Takeda S, et al: Leptin inhibits bone formation through a hypothalamic relay: a central control of bone mass. Cell 2000;100:197–207.
24 Hamrick MW, Pennington C, Newton D, Xie D, Isales C: Leptin deficiency produces contrasting phenotypes in bones of the limb and spine. Bone 2004;34:376–383.
25 Steppan CM, Crawford DT, Chidsey-Frink KL, Ke H, Swick AG: Leptin is a potent stimulator of bone growth in ob/ob mice. Regul Pept 2000;92:73–78.
26 Lu M, Tang Q, Olefsky JM, Mellon PL, Webster NJ: Adiponectin activates adenosine monophosphate-activated protein kinase and decreases luteinizing hormone secretion in LbetaT2 gonadotropes. Mol Endocrinol 2008;22:760–771.
27 Luo XH, Guo LJ, Xie H, et al: Adiponectin stimulates RANKL and inhibits OPG expression in human osteoblasts through the MAPK signaling pathway. J Bone Miner Res 2006;21:1648–1656.
28 Luo XH, Guo LJ, Yuan LQ, et al: Adiponectin stimulates human osteoblasts proliferation and differentiation via the MAPK signaling pathway. Exp Cell Res 2005;309:99–109.
29 Rodriguez-Pacheco F, Martinez-Fuentes AJ, Tovar S, et al: Regulation of pituitary cell function by adiponectin. Endocrinology 2007;148:401–410.
30 Fukushima N, Hanada R, Teranishi H, et al: Ghrelin directly regulates bone formation. J Bone Miner Res 2005;20:790–798.
31 Kluge M, Schussler P, Uhr M, Yassouridis A, Steiger A: Ghrelin suppresses secretion of luteinizing hormone in humans. J Clin Endocrinol Metab 2007;92:3202–3205.
32 Baldock PA, Sainsbury A, Couzens M, et al: Hypothalamic Y2 receptors regulate bone formation. J Clin Invest 2002;109:915–921.

33 Fernandez-Fernandez R, Aguilar E, Tena-Sempere M, Pinilla L: Effects of polypeptide YY(3–36) upon luteinizing hormone-releasing hormone and gonadotropin secretion in prepubertal rats: in vivo and in vitro studies. Endocrinology 2005;146:1403–1410.
34 Misra M, Miller KK, Tsai P, et al: Elevated peptide YY levels in adolescent girls with anorexia nervosa. J Clin Endocrinol Metab 2006;91:1027–1033.
35 Considine RV, Sinha MK, Heiman ML, et al: Serum immunoreactive-leptin concentrations in normal-weight and obese humans. N Engl J Med 1996;334: 292–295.
36 Kennedy A, Gettys TW, Watson P, et al: The metabolic significance of leptin in humans: gender-based differences in relationship to adiposity, insulin sensitivity, and energy expenditure. J Clin Endocrinol Metab 1997;82:1293–1300.
37 Saad MF, Riad-Gabriel MG, Khan A, et al: Diurnal and ultradian rhythmicity of plasma leptin: effects of gender and adiposity. J Clin Endocrinol Metab 1998;83:453–459.
38 Cambuli VM, Musiu MC, Incani M, et al: Assessment of adiponectin and leptin as biomarkers of positive metabolic outcomes after lifestyle intervention in overweight and obese children. J Clin Endocrinol Metab 2008;93:3051–3057.
39 Yang WS, Lee WJ, Funahashi T, et al: Weight reduction increases plasma levels of an adipose-derived anti-inflammatory protein, adiponectin. J Clin Endocrinol Metab 2001;86:3815–3819.
40 Misra M, Miller KK, Kuo K, et al: Secretory dynamics of leptin in adolescent girls with anorexia nervosa and healthy adolescents. Am J Physiol Endocrinol Metab 2005;289:E373–E381.
41 Farooqi IS: Leptin and the onset of puberty: insights from rodent and human genetics. Semin Reprod Med 2002;20:139–144.
42 Misra M, Miller KK, Cord J, et al: Relationships between serum adipokines, insulin levels, and bone density in girls with anorexia nervosa. J Clin Endocrinol Metab 2007;92:2046–2052.
43 Pannacciulli N, Bunt JC, Ortega E, et al: Lower total fasting plasma adiponectin concentrations are associated with higher metabolic rates. J Clin Endocrinol Metab 2006;91:1600–1603.
44 Gimble JM, Zvonic S, Floyd ZE, Kassem M, Nuttall ME: Playing with bone and fat. J Cell Biochem 2006;98:251–266.
45 Pei L, Tontonoz P: Fat's loss is bone's gain. J Clin Invest 2004;113:805–806.
46 Jurimae J, Rembel K, Jurimae T, Rehand M: Adiponectin is associated with bone mineral density in perimenopausal women. Horm Metab Res 2005;37: 297–302.
47 Lenchik L, Register TC, Hsu FC, et al: Adiponectin as a novel determinant of bone mineral density and visceral fat. Bone 2003;33:646–651.
48 Nakazato M, Murakami N, Date Y, et al: A role for ghrelin in the central regulation of feeding. Nature 2001;409:194–198.
49 Tschop M, Smiley DL, Heiman ML: Ghrelin induces adiposity in rodents. Nature 2000;407:908–913.
50 De Souza MJ, Leidy HJ, O'Donnell E, Lasley B, Williams NI: Fasting ghrelin levels in physically active women: relationship with menstrual disturbances and metabolic hormones. J Clin Endocrinol Metab 2004;89:3536–3542.
51 Jurimae J, Jurimae T, Purge P: Plasma ghrelin is altered after maximal exercise in elite male rowers. Exp Biol Med (Maywood) 2007;232:904–909.
52 Hotta M, Ohwada R, Katakami H, et al: Plasma levels of intact and degraded ghrelin and their responses to glucose infusion in anorexia nervosa. J Clin Endocrinol Metab 2004;89:5707–5712.
53 Misra M, Miller KK, Kuo K, et al: Secretory dynamics of ghrelin in adolescent girls with anorexia nervosa and healthy adolescents. Am J Physiol Endocrinol Metab 2005;289:E347–E356.
54 Vulliemoz NR, Xiao E, Xia-Zhang L, et al: Decrease in luteinizing hormone pulse frequency during a five-hour peripheral ghrelin infusion in the ovariectomized rhesus monkey. J Clin Endocrinol Metab 2004;89:5718–5723.
55 Kamegai J, Tamura H, Shimizu T, et al: Chronic central infusion of ghrelin increases hypothalamic neuropeptide Y and Agouti-related protein mRNA levels and body weight in rats. Diabetes 2001;50: 2438–2443.
56 Arvat E, Maccario M, Di Vito L, et al: Endocrine activities of ghrelin, a natural growth hormone secretagogue (GHS), in humans: comparison and interactions with hexarelin, a nonnatural peptidyl GHS, and GH-releasing hormone. J Clin Endocrinol Metab 2001;86:1169–1174.
57 Takaya K, Ariyasu H, Kanamoto N, et al: Ghrelin strongly stimulates growth hormone release in humans. J Clin Endocrinol Metab 2000;85:4908–4911.
58 Misra M, Miller KK, Stewart V, et al: Ghrelin and bone metabolism in adolescent girls with anorexia nervosa and healthy adolescents. J Clin Endocrinol Metab 2005;90:5082–5087.
59 Huda MS, Wilding JP, Pinkney JH: Gut peptides and the regulation of appetite. Obes Rev 2006;7:163–182.

60 Ballantyne GH: Peptide YY(1–36) and peptide YY(3–36). II. Changes after gastrointestinal surgery and bariatric surgery. Obes Surg 2006;16:795–803.
61 Keire DA, Mannon P, Kobayashi M, et al: Primary structures of PYY, [Pro(34)]PYY, and PYY-(3–36) confer different conformations and receptor selectivity. Am J Physiol Gastrointest Liver Physiol 2000; 279:G126–G131.
62 Batterham RL, Cohen MA, Ellis SM, et al: Inhibition of food intake in obese subjects by peptide YY3–36. N Engl J Med 2003;349:941–948.

Madhusmita Misra, MD, MPH
BUL 457, Neuroendocrine Unit
Massachusetts General Hospital
Boston, MA 02114 (USA)
Tel. +1 617 726 3870, Fax +1 617 726 8528, E-Mail mmisra@partners.org

Jürimäe J, Hills AP, Jürimäe T (eds): Cytokines, Growth Mediators and Physical Activity in Children during Puberty.
Med Sport Sci. Basel, Karger, 2010, vol 55, pp 114–127

Bone Turnover Markers during Pubertal Development: Relationships with Growth Factors and Adipocytokines

Jaak Jürimäe · Jarek Mäestu · Toivo Jürimäe

Institute of Sport Pedagogy and Coaching Sciences, Center of Behavioral and Health Sciences, University of Tartu, Tartu, Estonia

Abstract

The rapid increase in skeletal mass that occurs during puberty is caused by increases in longitudinal growth as well as cortical thickness. The measurement of growth changes during puberty using two-dimensional (dual-energy X-ray absorptiometry) and/or three-dimensional (computed tomography, magnetic resonance imaging) measurement devices provides only a static representation of bone tissue parameters. The measurement of bone turnover markers provides a more dynamic picture of the nature of bone tissue that can be repeated at much shorter intervals during puberty. The bone turnover markers are products of osteoblasts and osteoclasts which can be measured in urine or blood. The increase in different markers of bone turnover coincides with the pubertal growth spurt and thereafter markers decline until they converge into adult values. The initiation of puberty is accompanied by increases in androgens and estrogens. The effects of sex hormones on bone mineral accrual are mediated mainly by growth hormone and insulin-like growth factor-1, but they also exert a direct effect on bone metabolism. Important determinants of bone mineral accrual during puberty include optimal nutritional status, body composition parameters and physical activity pattern. All of these determinants are related to the state of energy balance, while peripheral indicators of energy balance, such as different growth factors and adipocytokines, may also have a positive influence of the growing skeleton. Taken together, bone mineral accrual during puberty is a complex interaction between physical activity pattern, various body composition parameters, specific growth factors and adipocytokines, and also sex hormones.

The pubertal years are an important period for linear growth and bone mineral accretion. Bone mineralization increases with age, height, and body mass throughout childhood, with a significant gain during pubertal development, resulting in an increase of bone mineral density (BMD) of about 40% during this period [1]. In a longitudinal study over 15 years in Canadian boys and girls, it was found that 8.3% of adult height and 22% of adult total body bone mineral content (BMC) was gained in the 2 years surrounding peak height velocity (PHV) [2]. However, the pubertal growth spurt varies considerably in timing, tempo and duration among individuals [3]. Bone mineral accrual during puberty is more dependent on sexual maturation than chronological age, and both androgens and estrogens promote the deposition of bone mineral [4]. Therefore, adolescents with delayed puberty or secondary amenorrhea may fail to accrue bone mineral normally, and consequently have reduced BMD as adults [5]. Estrogen levels make the greatest contribution to bone mineral accretion during puberty in boys and girls, while testosterone level makes only a modest contribution to the increase of BMD in boys [4].

Rising levels of estrogen in early puberty are followed closely by increasing growth hormone (GH) and insulin-like growth factor-1 (IGF-1) concentrations, both of which are important bone trophic hormones and important for pubertal bone modeling [6, 7]. Important determinants of bone mineral accrual during puberty are also optimal nutritional status [8], body composition parameters [6] and physical activity pattern [9]. Each of these determinants are related to the state of energy balance, and peripheral indicators of energy balance, such as different adipocytokines, may also have a positive influence on the BMD of the growing skeleton [10, 11]. It is well known that a critical amount of body fat is essential for the onset of puberty in females [12], and different adipocytokines and growth factors, including leptin and ghrelin, have been demonstrated to play a role in linear growth and pubertal timing [13, 14]. Specifically, the initiation of puberty has been linked to increased leptin [13] and decreased ghrelin [14] concentrations. Thus, it appears that bone mineral accrual in adolescents is dependent on multiple mechanical and biochemical factors which may impact on bone modelling of the growing bone. All of these factors need to be considered when assessing bone development during puberty.

Linear growth involves an orderly process of soft tissue synthesis, epiphyseal bone growth and extensive modeling in addition to remodeling [15]. However, the assessment of growth changes in these processes using two-dimensional (dual-energy X-ray absorptiometry; DXA) and/or three-dimensional (computed tomography, magnetic resonance imaging) measurement devices provides only a static representation of bone tissue parameters. The measurement of different bone turnover markers provides a more dynamic picture of the nature of bone tissue that can be repeated at much shorter intervals during pubertal development. Accordingly, the aim of this review is to discuss various bone turnover markers and to evaluate the influence of different growth factors and adipocytokines on these markers in children during pubertal development.

Bone Turnover Markers

Bone is a metabolically active tissue with continuous remodeling occurring across the lifespan. BMD is a result of the dynamic process of bone formation and bone resorption [16]. The dramatic accumulation of BMC during puberty is caused by changes in both modeling and remodeling during this period of life. The rapid increase in skeletal mass that occurs during puberty is caused by increases in both longitudinal growth as well as cortical thickness [17]. Accordingly, markers of bone turnover may not be easy to interpret in children as they are released into the circulation during the processes of bone modelling, remodeling, and growth in length [15, 17, 18]. Another limitation of using bone metabolism markers is that they represent an average of turnover from all skeletal sites in the body and consequently are not site-specific [16]. Nearly all bone turnover markers also demonstrate a diurnal variation with peak concentrations in the morning and a nadir in the late afternoon [19]. All of these factors should be taken into account when interpreting bone metabolism variables in maturing children.

Various molecular markers have been used to monitor bone growth in children during puberty (table 1). The bone turnover markers are products of osteoblasts and osteoclasts which can be measured in urine or blood [28]. Commonly used blood markers of bone formation are alkaline phosphatase (AP), bone-specific alkaline phosphatase (BAP), osteocalcin (OC), and procollagen type 1 propeptides, carboxy-terminal (PICP) and amino-terminal (PINP), which are released at different stages of osteoblast proliferation and differentiation [21, 23, 28]. The bone resorption markers are either degradation products of bone type 1 collagen, or the osteoclast-specific enzyme tartrate-resistant acid phosphatase (TRACP) [28]. Among others, the commonly used marker of bone resorption is type 1 cross-linked N-telopeptide (NTX), which solely originates from type 1 collagen in the bone by osteoclast activity and can be measured in urine and serum [18]. Other commonly used degradation products of type 1 collagen are type 1 cross-linked C-telopeptide (CTX) measured in urine and serum, and urinary markers pyridioline (PYR) and deoxypyridinoline (DPD) [28]. In addition, a serum marker of collagen type 1 cross-linked C-terminal telopeptide generated by matrix metalloproteinases (ICTP) has been measured to assess bone resorption in children [15].

It has been suggested that the increase in different markers of bone turnover coincides with the pubertal growth spurt [15, 18, 23]. For example, van Coeverden et al. [23] found that ICTP is a good marker for BMC and for BMC increment as well as for height and height velocity, compared to other markers of bone formation and bone resorption, during pubertal growth spurt in boys. Puberty is related to a relative increase in bone degradation rates [29], but bone formation exceeds bone resorption [23]. Blumsohn et al. [20] reported the highest levels of bone turnover markers in pubertal stages 2 and 3 in girls, while van der Sluis et al. [18] found that the peak concentrations of different bone turnover markers occurred at the age of 12 years in girls and approximately 2.5 years later in boys. In another study, Mora et al. [30] found peak values for bone turnover markers in early puberty (pubertal stage 2) with the lowest values in the later stages of puberty in boys and girls. Our recent study also demonstrated highest values for PINP and ICTP in boys at pubertal stages 2

Table 1. Commonly measured bone turnover markers children and adolescents, and the supporting evidence for increases in these markers during puberty

Bone turnover marker	Acronyms[1]	Studies with increased bone turnover markers during puberty
Bone formation marker		
Alkaline phosphatase	AP	[17,18,20,20–23]
Bone-specific alkaline phosphatase	BAP	[15,21,23,24]
Osteocalcin	OC	[15,17,18,21–23,25]
Procollagen type 1 C-terminal propeptide	PICP	[20–22]
Procollagen type 1 N-terminal propeptide	PINP	[6,18,21,23,26,27]
Bone resorption marker		
Pyridinoline[2]	PYD	[17,20]
Deoxypyridinoline[2]	DPD	[17,20,23]
Collagen type 1 cross-linked N-terminal telopeptide	NTX	[6,18,22,27]
Collagen type 1 cross-linked C-terminal telopeptide	CTX	[15,18,24]
Collagen type 1 cross-linked C-terminal telopeptide generated by matrix metalloproteinases	ICTP	[15,18,23,26]
Tartrade-resistant acid phosphatase (isoenzyme 5b)	TRACP	[15,25]

[1] The acronyms are not standard, the most used acronyms also used in the present paper have been reported.
[2] These markers are generally known as pyridinium cross-links or simply cross-links.

and 3 in comparison with prepubertal boys (pubertal stage 1) and boys at pubertal stages 4 and 5 [26]. However, some investigations have suggested that peak values for bone turnover markers are achieved later in puberty (pubertal stage 4) [23]. Bone formation and bone resorption markers demonstrate a good relationship with growth velocity [15, 23]. In the period of growth spurt until PHV, increases of bone turnover and bone longitudinal growth as well as BMC are high. The maximum height velocity is reached at an early stage in girls (pubertal stage 3) compared to boys (pubertal stage 4) [23]. However, in the period after PHV when height velocity declines, bone mineral accrual still increases [23, 31]. Bailey [31] demonstrated that the peak velocity in bone mass accumulation occurred 0.7 years after PHV. Accordingly, bone mineral accrual has been found to be greatest at pubertal stage 4 in boys or at menarche in girls (pubertal stage 2 or 3) [18, 23, 32]. Typically, concentrations of most bone turnover markers increase from prepuberty to mid-puberty and decline during late puberty with the lowest values in the transition to adulthood [4, 15, 23, 26]. Because growth and puberty are usually completed by late adolescence, markers of bone formation and bone resorption converge into adult values [19].

Bone formation and bone resorption markers have usually been reported to correlate well with each other at all pubertal stages [18, 23, 26]. This is expected as bone turnover is a strongly coupled mechanism of bone resorption by osteoclasts and bone formation by osteoblasts. However, Rauchenzauner et al. [15] found only weak associations among different markers of bone formation and bone resorption in boys at different pubertal stages. In addition, it has been reported that low concentrations of bone formation and bone resorption markers predict increased BMD values in children during the development of peak skeletal mass [25]. Significant negative associations between bone turnover markers (PINP and ICTP) and lumbar spine bone mineral apparent density (BMAD) have been found in boys at different stages of biological maturation [26]. These results together suggest that bone turnover markers are informative for monitoring bone development in maturing children during puberty.

Bone Turnover and Physical Activity

Physical activity is known to induce modifications in BMD [9] and bone turnover [6, 33] values in adolescents. The specific mechanisms by which bone metabolism is influenced by physical activity are still not thoroughly understood. There are very few data regarding bone turnover markers in adolescent athletes. Mechanical loading in athletes and associated bone modeling and remodeling should be associated with increased levels of bone turnover markers [7]. Indeed, female athletes involved in high-impact sports such as basketball and volleyball displayed higher levels of serum OC, a bone formation marker, and higher BMDs at weight-bearing sites compared to athletes participating in a nonimpact sport (swimming) and control subjects [16]. In another study, higher levels of serum OC were reported in adolescent athletes compared to adult athletes [34], which is consistent with the increased state of bone turnover in the adolescent years [7].

In a recent study with adolescent athletes, a lower level of bone formation (PINP) and bone resorption (NTX) markers was observed in adolescent athletes with amenorrhea compared with sedentary controls, whereas levels in athletes with eumenorrhea were somewhere in between [6]. This finding was unexpected, given that BMD was slightly greater in eumenorrheic athletes compared to the other two groups, leading to expectations of higher levels of bone formation and lower levels of bone resorption markers in athletes with eumenorrhea [6]. The lower levels of bone turnover markers in eumenorrheic athletes were explained by somewhat lower levels of growth factors in these athletes [6]. In addition, bone age was the strongest predictor of bone turnover markers in these female adolescent athletes, and girls with greater bone age had lower levels of bone turnover markers [6]. This is in accordance with the decreases in bone turnover seen in late adolescence when little growth potential remains [7]. However, another study with adolescent male athletes found that those in the high impact load group (gymnastics, athletics, basketball and tennis) presented higher values for all BMD measurements. In contrast, athletes in the active load group (swimming and water polo) had higher values for bone formation (BAP) and bone resorption (DPD) markers and lower values for testosterone [35]. It was suggested that adolescent athletes involved in non-weight-bearing exercise regimens may have a delay in bone growth acquisition compared to athletes involved in weight-bearing exercise [35]. Lima et al. [35] argued that the significant difference in testosterone levels between groups is suggestive of the involvement of this hormone in bone acquisition in adolescent male athletes. In summary, few studies have examined bone mass accrual together with bone turnover markers over time in athletes. It is important to determine whether bone development is affected by athletic activity and environmental influences during puberty.

The only longitudinal study with adolescent athletes was undertaken by Eliakim et al. [33]. Thirty-eight healthy males (15–17 years of age) participated in a 5-week programme in which one group of participants was assigned to a training condition consisting of a 2-hour daily endurance training programme five times a week, and the group represented the control condition without physical activity. Training resulted in an increase in bone formation (OC, BAP, PICP) and a decrease in bone resorption (NTX) markers. These bone turnover markers did not change in control participants and there was no change DPD and CTX in either group [33]. Accordingly, it was concluded that a relatively brief period of endurance training stimulates bone formation in adolescent males [33].

Relationship of Growth Factors with Bone Metabolism Values

The initiation of puberty is accompanied by an increase in sex hormones [11, 23]. However, the effects of sex hormones on bone are mediated mainly by GH and IGF-I [36], but they also exert a direct effect on bone metabolism [23, 26, 37]. In early puberty, bone development is stimulated by low levels of circulating sex hormones in combination with increasing levels of GH and IGF-1 [23]. Both estrogens and androgens have been shown to stimulate the proliferation of osteoblasts [38]. In our recent study, the positive associations of testosterone with bone formation (PINP) and bone resorption (ICTP) markers were observed in early puberty (pubertal stages 2 and

3) but disappeared in late puberty (pubertal stages 4 and 5) [26] similar to previous investigations [23]. It remains unclear whether these associations were caused by the effect of testosterone itself or that of estrogens aromatized from testosterone. No correlation between testosterone and bone formation markers (BAP, OC) during puberty was observed in a study Yilmaz et al. [4]. Accordingly, estrogen makes the greatest contribution to bone mineral acquisition during puberty [4, 23, 28]. Male patients with either estrogen receptor deficiency or aromatase deficiency have reduced BMD and absence of a pubertal growth spurt [39]. However, Riis et al. [40] reported that direct or indirect acute stimulation of bone formation by an increase in testosterone concentrations during puberty is followed by a highly significant increase in BMC in boys. Similarly, testosterone concentration was strongly associated with measured BMD parameters in boys during pubertal development [4, 37]. These results indicate that testosterone may stimulate bone formation markers at the initiation of puberty in boys. However, a significant negative correlation between bone turnover markers and estrogen concentration in late puberty in girls suggests that high levels of estradiol could contribute to the reduction of bone turnover in late puberty [4, 20]. This leads to a decline in height velocity and an immediate decline of bone formation and bone resorption markers [23]. The dramatic decrease in bone turnover markers observed after puberty in both sexes probably reflects bone formation and bone resorption inhibition by estrogen [23, 24].

IGF-1 is an important regulator of bone turnover at the tissue level. It has been shown to enhance osteoblast proliferation, to stimulate type 1 collagen production and to modulate osteoblast-ostoeclast interactions [24]. Most GH anabolic actions on bone are also mediated through IGF-1 [41]. The role of IGF-1 in bone mineralization is particularly important around the age of 13–14 years when the pubertal growth spurt should reach its peak [37, 42]. The positive associations between IGF-1 and bone turnover markers have been reported during all pubertal stages [23] however, it has also been reported that the positive associations that exist between IGF-1 and bone turnover markers in prepuberty and early puberty (pubertal stages 2 and 3) may disappear in late puberty (pubertal stages 4 and 5) [24]. The absence of a strong relationship during late puberty may be related to major changes in circulating estrogen, testosterone and aromatized testosterone levels, and in interactions between sex hormones and the GH-IGF-1 system, bone turnover and growth [24, 38]. In another study, IGF-1 concentration correlated with bone formation marker (PINP) in the whole group of adolescent female participants while low levels of IGF-1 were not related to PINP values in adolescent female athletes with amenorrhea [6]. Estrogen has an important effect on bone mass acquisition in adolescence and prolonged hypoestrogenism together with low IGF-1 levels and associated low energy availability during this period, could have serious implications for peak BMC in adolescent female athletes with amenorrhea [6, 7]. Furthermore, a strong relationship between the magnitude of reduction in IGF-1 concentration and markers of bone formation has been observed under the conditions of energy restriction in female endurance runners [43]. These results would suggest that inadequate energy balance may also have an effect on bone development in adolescent female athletes.

An elevated energy expenditure as a result of childhood athletic activity may cause a decreased energy balance and have a negative influence on bone mineralization [7]. The orexigenic hormone ghrelin has been implicated to influence energy homeostasis [7, 44] and also bone metabolism [8, 45]. It has been reported that ghrelin could influence growth and physical development [14]. However, the evidence is limited regarding the exact role of ghrelin on bone mineral accrual during puberty. While sex hormones induce pubertal growth at least partly by influencing GH release [23], ghrelin is also known to influence GH release in response to changes in energy homeostasis [46]. Furthermore, it has been demonstrated that testosterone is negatively related to ghrelin concentration in boys at different maturational levels [47]. These assumptions, together with the evidence that GH stimulates bone formation [4], raised the possibility that ghrelin may play a role in bone metabolism during puberty. In addition, an in vitro study demonstrated that ghrelin administration increased osteoblast proliferation and differentiation in cell culture [48]. In contrast, no relationship between ghrelin concentration and markers of bone turnover at different stages of pubertal development has been found in boys [26]. These results are in accordance with the results of previous cross-sectional studies with physically inactive boys at different maturational levels [11, 37]. Our recent longitudinal study with athletes also demonstrated that ghrelin was not related to measured BMD values, nor were year-to-year changes in ghrelin concentration related to changes in measured BMD values throughout the pubertal development in young male competitive swimmers [49]. However, the relatively high ghrelin concentrations caused by elevated energy expenditure in athletes may explain why no relationship between circulating ghrelin and measured bone mineral variables was observed [49]. In contrast, significant relationships between ghrelin and measured BMD variables were observed in trained boys at different maturation levels [11]. Other studies have also demonstrated that ghrelin levels are related to bone mineralization in healthy adolescent girls [8] and in obese and normal-weight children and adolescent groups of both sexes [45].

It has been suggested that the role of ghrelin in bone development is largely mediated through testosterone and explains independently only a small fraction of the variability in bone mineral parameters [37]. For example, in a multiple regression analysis, ghrelin was an important determinant of BMD parameters in boys only after removal of testosterone [37]. It is interesting to note that a significant negative correlation between ghrelin and testosterone levels was observed only after the evolution of puberty (i.e. pubertal stages 2 and 3) [47]. In accordance with these results, we found that changes in circulating ghrelin were also related to changes in testosterone only after the evolution of puberty in male athletes [49]. These results together suggest that the role of ghrelin in bone development may be largely mediated through testosterone during pubertal development and ghrelin has no direct influence on bone metabolism markers in boys [26, 49]. However, further longitudinal studies together with different bone formation and bone resorption markers are warranted to further clarify the role of ghrelin in bone metabolism during biological maturation.

Relationships of Adipocytokines with Bone Metabolism Values

The effect of body mass on bone turnover and bone mineral variables is probably contributed by both fat mass (FM) and fat-free mass (FFM), though FM has been more consistently demonstrated to be important [50]. A number of mechanisms exist for the fat-bone relationship and include the effect of FM on skeletal loading, the association of FM with the secretion of bone active hormones from the pancreatic beta cell, and the secretion of bone active hormones from the adipocyte [50, 51]. Adipose tissue is now considered as an endocrine organ that produces many adipocytokines which participate in bone metabolism [50, 51]. Leptin, the product of the LEP gene, has been regarded as the classic adipocyte hormone that can directly modulate the activity of bone cells, as well as indirectly influence skeletal metabolism through its actions on the central nervous system [50, 51]. Peripherally, leptin is thought to exert positive effects on bone formation and bone resorption, whilst it has been associated with a reduction in bone turnover via a central control mechanism when acting directly on the hypothalamus [50, 51]. However, descriptions of the effect of leptin on bone metabolism markers in humans are very limited [50]. Despite the observation of the positive effect of leptin on bone mineral variables in the growing skeleton in healthy prepubertal children [10], results regarding the role of leptin in more mature bone have been conflicting [51]. Courteix et al. [52] found that hypoleptinemia induced by intensive and stressful physical training did not affect bone health in elite adolescent rhythmic gymnasts. This may suggest that weight-bearing exercises are more important determinants of bone health than body composition variables in adolescent elite athletes. In contrast, leptin concentrations were inversely related to bone resorption markers in young adult athletes [53]. Proteau et al. [53] examined the relationship between circulating leptin concentration with bone formation (OC) and bone resorption (CTX) markers and body composition in female judoists during stable body mass, in response to body mass reduction and also to body mass regain. The negative association between leptin and CTX was observed at stable body mass and also in response to body mass loss and regain. Therefore, the bone formation marker (OC) remained unaffected by body mass reduction and following regain in young female athletes [53]. A 3-month leptin treatment program in women with hypothalamic amenorrhea resulted in significantly increased bone formation markers (BAP, OC) together with increased estradiol and IGF-I concentrations, which demonstrated different indirect mechanisms by which leptin can impact bone tissue [54]. However, another study found that leptin secretion did not predict BMD in adolescent athletes with amenorrhea [7].

Typically, both circulating leptin concentrations and bone mineral increase at the initiation of puberty [13, 55]. These relationships have led to the suggestion that leptin may modulate bone mineral accrual but the exact mechanism still remains unclear [56]. For example, evidence for a stimulatory role of leptin on bone mineralization includes associations of leptin concentrations with BMC and BMD values in lean prepubertal and pubertal boys and girls [10, 56]. However, rather weak relationships and incomplete control for potential confounding factors may have influenced these results [56]. In another study, Roemmich et al. [56] demonstrated that in normal-weight children and adolescents across all pubertal stages, leptin concentrations were not related to total body nor regional BMC and BMD independent of chronological age, FM, bone-free FFM, and circulating estradiol and IGF-1 concentrations. Accordingly, it appears that leptin does not increase bone mineral accrual beyond the biomechanical influence of body mass and physiological influences of FM, sex steroids, and the GH-IGF-1 axis in children during puberty [56]. However, there is a need for longitudinal studies together with bone turnover markers to determine the exact role of leptin on bone mineral accrual during pubertal development in children before any conclusions can be drawn.

Among others, adiponectin is an adipose tissue-derived hormone that may have a role in bone metabolism [50, 51]. An inverse association between adiponectin and BMD in adult [57, 58] and also adolescent [59] females has been reported. However, the relationship between adiponectin and BMD was no longer significant after adjustment for FM and pubertal stage in this group [59]. Recently, Russell et al. [27] found that circulating adiponectin concentration did not contribute to hypogonadism and impaired bone metabolism in adolescent amenorrheic female athletes with decreased energy availability. Specifically, adiponectin concentration was not independently related to estradiol, and lumbar spine BMAD, bone formation (PINP) and bone resoprtion (NTX) markers. In addition, adiponectin levels were also not different between adolescent amenorrheic and eumenorrheic athletes [27]. Adiponectin and its receptors are expressed in osteoblasts and osteoclasts [50, 51] and the negative effect of adiponectin on BMD may be mediated by the promotion of bone resorption [60]. Further studies with adipenectin and different bone turnover markers in children at different maturational levels should be conducted to understand the possible role of adiponectin in bone mineral accrual during puberty, taking into account that pubertal development influences adiponectin levels in boys but not in girls [61, 62].

Resistin, tumor-necrosis factor-α (TNF-α) and interleukin-6 (IL-6) have also been found to mediate bone metabolism [50, 51]. Resistin is expressed in osteoblasts and osteoclasts [63] and has been found to be a significant negative predictor of lumbar spine BMD in humans [64]. TNF-α and IL-6 have been shown to stimulate bone resorption [50, 51]. Circulating levels of IL-6 have been reported to correlate negatively with BMC in girls at pubertal stages 3 and 4 [17]. IL-6 concentrations decrease during pubertal development in both sexes [62] and IL-6 may be involved in mediating decreased bone resorption during late puberty [17]. However, further investigations are warranted to detail the role of sex hormone-induced inhibition of production of IL-6 and other adipocytokines in mediating reduced bone turnover and increased bone mineral development during puberty [17].

Conclusions and Future Research

The rapid increase in skeletal mass that occurs during puberty is caused by increases in both longitudinal growth as well as cortical thickness. Bone mineral development during puberty is more dependent on sexual maturation than chronological age. Bone mineral accrual during puberty is a complex interaction among specific mechanical loading and physical activity patterns, different body composition parameters, specific growth factors, and also sex hormones. The influence of energy availability, together with reproductive function on bone mineral accrual during puberty, is also important to consider. The inadequate caloric intake and hypogonadism often associated with adolescent athletic activity exposes young female athletes to several health risks including negative effects on the development of BMD. As DXA measurement of BMD only represents a static assessment of bone health, the more dynamic nature of the bone development can be obtained by measuring biochemical markers of bone formation and bone resorption in blood and/or urine. It has been suggested that the increase in different bone turnover markers coincides with the pubertal growth spurt. Furthermore, it has been found that different bone formation and bone resorption markers peak at pubertal stages 2 and 3, and thereafter decline until they converge into adult values. In early puberty, estrogen and testosterone together with IGF-1 mostly stimulate bone turnover markers, while ghrelin and adipocytokines have no direct influence on bone turnover markers. The effects of ghrelin and adipocytokines on bone mineral accrual may depend on specific body composition, sex hormone, and GH-IGF-1 axis parameters in children during puberty. However, to our knowledge, no longitudinal studies have investigated bone mineral accrual throughout puberty measuring bone formation and resorption markers together with body composition, physical activity, sex hormones, growth factors and adipocytokines.

The skeleton has also recently been recognized as an endocrine organ [51]. The participation of adipocytokines in the regulation of bone remodeling has led to the hypothesis that bone may exert a role in the feedback control of energy homeostasis [65]. It has been suggested that bone-derived factors (osteokines) exert an endocrine regulation on glucose homeostasis and body mass [51]. These findings expand the biological importance of the skeleton and our understanding of energy metabolism. It could be speculated that osteokine levels in blood could be used to characterize energy balance in children during biological maturation. Accordingly, it is important to measure bone turnover markers when studying interactions between adipose and bone tissues during pubertal development in children.

References

1 Gordon CL, Halton JM, Atkinson SA: The contributions of growth and puberty to peak bone mass. Growth Dev Aging 1991;55:257–262.

2 Bailey DA, Faulkner RA, Mirwald RL, Sherar L, Baxter-Jones AGD: Bone mineral accrual over 15 years from pre-adolescence into adulthood. J Bone Miner Res 2006;21:S30.

3 Malina RM, Bouchard C, Bar-Or O: Growth, Maturation, and Physical Activity. Champaign, Human Kinetics. 2004.

4 Yilmaz D, Ersoy B, Bilgin E, Gümüser G, Onur E, Pinar ED: Bone mineral density in girls and boys at different pubertal stages: relation with gonadal steroids, bone formation markers, and growth parameters. J Bone Miner Metab 2005;23:476–482.

5 Slemenda CW, Reister TK, Hui SL, Miller JZ, Christian JC, Johnston CC: Influence of skeletal mineralization in children and adolescents: evidence for varying effects of sexual maturation and physical activity. J Pediatr 1994;125:201–207.

6 Christo K, Prabhakaran R, Lamparello B, Cord J, Miller KK, Goldstein MA, Gupta N, Herzog DB, Klibanski A, Misra M: Bone metabolism in adolescent athletes with amenorrhea, athletes with eumenorrhea, and control subjects. Pediatrics 2008;121: 1127–1136.

7 Misra M: Bone density in the adolescent athlete. Rev Endocr Metab Disord 2008;9:139–144.

8 Misra M, Miller KK, Stewart V, Hunter E, Kuo K, Herzog DB, Klibanski A: Ghrelin and bone metabolism in adolescent girls with anorexia nervosa and healthy adolescents. J Clin Endocrinol Metab 2005; 90:5082–5087.

9 Gruodyte R, Jürimäe J, Saar M, Jürimäe T: The relationships among bone health, insulin-like growth factor-1 and sex hormones in adolescent female athletes. J Bone Miner Metab 2010;28:306–313.

10 Garnett SP, Högler W, Blades B, Baur LA, Peat J, Lee J, Cowell CT: Relation between hormones and body composition, including bone, in prepubertal children. Am J Clin Nutr 2004;80:966–972.

11 Jürimäe J, Cicchella A, Tillmann V, Lätt E, Haljaste K, Purge P, Pomerants T, Jürimäe T: Effect of pubertal development and physical activity on plasma ghrelin concentration in boys. J Endocrinol Invest 2009;32:18–22.

12 Weise M, Eisenhofer G, Merke DP: Pubertal and gender-related changes in the sympathoadrenal system in healthy children. J Clin Endocrinol Metab 2002;87:5038–5043.

13 Clayton PE, Gill MS, Hall CM, Tillmann V, Whatmore AJ, Price DA: Serum leptin through childhood and adolescence. Clin Endocrinol 1997;46:727–733.

14 Whatmore AJ, Hall CM, Jones J, Westwood M, Clayton PE: Ghrelin concentrations in healthy children and adolescents. Clin Endocrinol 2003;59:649–654.

15 Rauchenzauner M, Schmid A, Heinz-Erian P, Kapelari K, Falkensammer G, Griesmacher A, Finkenstedt, Högler W: Sex- and age-specific reference curves for serum markers of bone turnover in healthy children from 2 months to 18 years. J Clin Endocrinol Metab 2007;92:443–449.

16 Creighton DL, Morgan AL, Boardley D, Brolinson PG: Weight-bearing exercise and markers of bone turnover in female athletes. Med Sci Sports Exerc 2001;90:565–570.

17 Libanti C, Baylink DJ, Lois-Wenzel E, Srinivasan N, Mohan S: Studies on the potential mediators of skeletal changes occurring during puberty in girls. J Clin Endocrinol Metab 1999;84:2807–2814.

18 van der Sluis IM, Hop WC, van Leeuwen JPTM, Pols HAP, de Muinck Keizer-Schrama SMPF: A cross-sectional study on biochemical parameters of bone turnover and vitamin D metabolites in healthy Dutch children and young adults. Horm Res 2002; 57:170–179.

19 Saggese G, Baroncelli GI, Bertelloni S, Cinquanta L, di Nero G: Twenty-four-hour osteocalcin, carboxyterminal propeptide of type I procollagen, and aminoterminal propeptide of type III procollagen rhythms in normal and growth-retarded children. Pediatr Res 1994;35:409–415.

20 Blumsohn A, Hannon RA, Wrate R, Barton J, Al-Dehaimi AW, Colwell A, Eastell R: Biochemical markers of bone turnover in girls during puberty. Clin Endocrinol 1994;40:663–670.

21 Magnusson P, Hager A, Larsson L: Serum osteocalcin and bone and liver alkaline phosphatase isoforms in healthy children and adolescents. Pediatr Res 1995;38:955–961.

22 Szulc P, Seeman E, Delmas PD: Biochemical measurements of bone turnover in children and adolescents. Osteoporos Int 2000;11:281–294.

23 van Coeverden SCCM, Netelenbos JC, de Ridder CM, Roos JC, Popp-Snijders C, Delemarre-van de Waal HA: Bone metabolism markers and bone mass in healthy pubertal boys and girls. Clin Endocrinol 2002;57:107–116.

24 Leger J, Mercat I, Alberti C, Chevenne D, Armoogum P, Tichet J, Czernichow P: The relationship between the GH/IGF-I axis and serum markers of bone turnover metabolism in healthy children. Eur J Endocrinol 2007;157:685–692.

25 Slemenda CW, Peacock M, Hui S, Zhou F, Johnston CC: Reduced rates of skeletal remodeling are associated with increased bone mineral density during the development of peak bone mass. J Bone Miner Res 1997;12:676–682.
26 Jürimäe J, Pomerants T, Tillmann V, Jürimäe T: Bone metabolism markers and ghrelin in boys at different stages of sexual maturity. Acta Paediatr 2009;98:892–896.
27 Russell M, Stark J, Nayak S, Miller KK, Herzog DB, Klibanski A, Misra M: Peptide YY in adolescent athletes with amenorrhea, eumenorrheic athletes and non-athletic controls. Bone 2009;45:104–109.
28 Eastell R: Role of oestrogen in the regulation of bone turnover at the menarche. J Endocrinol 2005; 185:223–234.
29 Conti A, Ferrero S, Giambona S, Sartorio A: Urinary free deoxypyridinoline levels during childhood. J Endocrinol Invest 1998;21:318–322.
30 Mora S, Pitukcheewanont P, Kaufman FR, Nelson JC, Gilsanz V: Biochemical markers of bone turnover and the volume and the density of bone in children at different stages of sexual development. J Bone Miner Res 1999;14:1664–1671.
31 Bailey DA: The Saskatchewan pediatric bone mineral accrual study: bone mineral acquisition during the growing years. Int J Sports Med 1997;18: S191–S194.
32 Theintz G, Buchs B, Rizzoli R, Slosman D, Clavien H, Sizonenko PC, Bonjour JP: Longitudinal monitoring of bone mass accumulation in healthy adolescents: evidence for a marked reduction after 16 years of age at the levels of lumbar spine and femoral neck in female subjects. J Clin Endocrinol Metab 1992;75:1060–1065.
33 Eliakim A, Raisz LG, Brasel JA, Cooper DM: Evidence for increased bone formation following a brief endurance-type training intervention in adolescent males. J Bone Miner Res 1997;12:1708–1713.
34 Kaga M, Takahashi K, Ishihara T, Suzuki H, Tanaka H, Seino Y, Makino H: Bone assessment of female long-distance runners. J Bone Miner Metab 2004;22: 509–513.
35 Lima F, de Falco V, Baima J, Carazzato JG, Pereira RMR: Effect of impact load and active load on bone metabolism and body composition of adolescent athletes. Med Sci Sports Exerc 2001;33:1318–1323.
36 Clark PA, Rogol AD: Growth hormones and sex steroid interactions at puberty. Endocrinol Metab Clin N Am 1996;25:665–681.
37 Pomerants T, Tillmann V, Jürimäe J, Jürimäe T: The influence of serum ghrelin, IGF axis and testosterone on bone mineral density in boys at different stages of sexual maturity. J Bone Miner Metab 2007; 25:193–197.
38 Veldhuis JD, Roemnich JN, Richmond EJ, Rogol AD, Lovejoy JC, Sheffield-Moore M, Mauras N, Bowers CY: Endocrine control of body composition in infancy, childhood, and puberty. Endocr Rev 2005;26:114–146.
39 Morishima A, Grumbach MM, Simpson ER, Fisher C, Qin K: Aromatase deficiency in male and female siblings caused by a novel mutation and the physiological role of estrogens. J Clin Endocrinol Metab 1995;80:3689–3698.
40 Riis BJ, Krabbe S, Christiansen C, Catherwood BD, Deftos LJ: Bone turnover in male puberty: a longitudinal study. Calcif Tissue Int 1985;37:213–217.
41 Patel MB, Arden NK, Masterson LM, Phillips DI, Swaminathan R, Syddall HE, Byrne CD, Wood PJ, Cooper C, Holt RI: Investigating the role of the growth hormone-insulin-like growth factor (GH-IHGF) axis as a determinant of male bone mineral density (BD). Bone 2005;37:833–841.
42 Kanbur NO, Derman O, Kinik E: The relationships between pubertal development, IGF-1 axis, and bone formation in healthy adolescents. J Bone Miner Metab 2005;23:76–83.
43 Zanker CL, Swane IL: Responses of bone turnover markers to repeated endurance running under conditions of energy balance or energy restriction. Eur J Appl Physiol 2000;83:434–440.
44 Jürimäe J, Cicchella A, Jürimäe T, Lätt E, Haljaste K, Purge P, Hamra J, von Duvillard SP: Regular physical activity influences plasma ghrelin concentration in adolescent girls. Med Sci Sports Exerc 2007;39: 1736–1741.
45 Pacifico L, Anania C, Poggiogalle E, Osborn JF, Prossomariti G, Martino F, Chiesa C: Relationships of acylated and des-acyl ghrelin levels to bone mineralization in obese children and adolescents. Bone 2009;45:274–279.
46 Wren AM, Small CJ, Ward HJ, Murphy KG, Dakin CL, Taheri S, Kennedy AR, Roberts GH, Morgan DG, Ghatei MA, Bloom SR: The novel hypothalamic peptide ghrelin stimulates food intake and growth hormone secretion. Endocrinology 2000; 141:4325–4328.
47 Pomerants T, Tillmann V, Jürimäe J, Jürimäe T: Relationship between ghrelin and anthropometrical, body composition parameters and testosterone levels in boys at different stages of puberty. J Endocrinol Invest 2006;29:962–967.
48 Maccarinelli G, Sibilia V, Torsello A, Raimondo F, Pitto M, Giustina A, Netti C, Cocchi D: Ghrelin regulates proliferation and differentation of osteoblastic cells. J Endocrinol 2005;184:249–256.
49 Jürimäe J, Lätt E, Haljaste K, Purge P, Cicchella A, Jürimäe T: Influence of puberty on ghrelin and BMD in athletes. Int J Sports Med 2009;30:403–407.

50 Reid IR: Relationships between fat and bone. Osteoporos Int 2008;19:595–606.
51 Gomez-Ambrosi J, Rodriguez A, Catalan V, Frühbeck G: The bone-adipose axis and weight loss. Obes Surg 2008;18:1134–1143.
52 Courteix D, Rieth N, Thomas T, van Praagh E, Benhamou CL, Collomp K, Lespessailles E, Jaffre C: Preserved bone health in adolescent elite rhythmic gymnasts despite hypoleptinemia. Horm Res 2007; 68:20–27.
53 Proteau S, Benhamou L, Courteix D: Relationships between serum leptin and bone markers during stable weight, weight reduction and weight regain in male and female judoists. Eur J Endocrinol 2006; 154:389–395.
54 Welt CK, Chan JL, Bullen J, Murphy R, Smith P, DePaoli AM, Karalis A, Mantzoros CS: Recombinant human leptin in women with hypothalamic amenorrhea. N Eng J Med 2004;351:987–997.
55 Mantzoros CS, Flier JS, Rogol AD: A longitudinal assessment of hormonal and physical alterations during normal puberty in boys. V. Rising leptin levels may signal the onset of puberty. J Clin Endocrinol Metab 1997;82:1066–1070.
56 Roemmich JN, Clark PA, Mantzoros CS, Gurgol CM, Weltman A, Rogol AD: Relationship of leptin to bone mineralization in children and adolescents. J Clin Endocrinol Metab 2003;88:599–604.
57 Jürimäe J, Jürimäe T: Adiponectin is a predictor of bone mineral density in middle-aged premenopausal women. Osteoporos Int 2007;18:1253–1259.
58 Richards JB, Valdes AM, Burling K, Perks UC, Spector TD: Serum adiponectin and bone mineral density in women. J Clin Endocrinol Metab 2007; 92:1517–1523.
59 Huang KC, Cheng WC, Yen RF, Tsai KS, Tui TY, Yang WS: Lack of independent relationship between plasma adiponectin, leptin levels and bone density in nondiabetic female adolescents. Clin Endocrinol 2004;61:204–208.
60 Peng XD, Xie H, Zhao Q, Wu XP, Sun ZQ, Liao EY: Relationships between serum adiponectin, leptin, resistin, visfatin levels and bone mineral density, and bone biochemical markers in Chinese men. Clin Chim Acta 2008;387:31–35.
61 Bottner A, Kratzsch J, Muller G, Kapellen TM, Bluher S, Keller E, Bluher M, Kiess W: Gender differences of adiponectin levels develop during the progression of puberty and are related to serum androgen levels. J Clin Endocrinol Metab 2004;89: 4053–4061.
62 Martos-Moreno GA, Barrios V, Argente J: Normative data for adiponectin, resistin, interleukin-6, and leptin/receptor ratio in a healthy Spanish pediatric population: relationship with sex steroids. Eur J Endocrinol 2006;155:429–434.
63 Thommesen L, Stunes AK, Monjo M, Grosvik K, Tamburstuen MV, Kjobli E, Lyngstadaas SP, Reseland JE, Syversen U: Expression and regulation of resistin in osteoblasts and osteoclasts indicate a role in bone metabolism. J Cell Biochem 2006;99:824–834.
64 Oh KW, Lee WY, Rhee EJ: The relationship between serum resistin, leptin, adiponectin, ghrelin levels and bone mineral density in middle-aged men. Clin Endocrinol 2005;63:131–138.
65 Lee NK, Sowa H, Hinoi E, Ferron M, Ahn JD, Confavreux C, Dacquin R, Mee PJ, McKee MD, Dung DJ, Zhang Z, Kim JK, Mauvais-Jarvis F, Ducy P, Karsenty G: Endocrine regulation of energy metabolism by the skeleton. Cell 2007;130:409–411.

Professor Jaak Jürimäe, PhD
Institute of Sport Pedagogy and Coaching Sciences, University of Tartu
18 Ülikooli Street
Tartu 50090 (Estonia)
Tel. +372 7 375372, Fax +372 7 375373, E-Mail jaakj@ut.ee

Jürimäe J, Hills AP, Jürimäe T (eds): Cytokines, Growth Mediators and Physical Activity in Children during Puberty.
Med Sport Sci. Basel, Karger, 2010, vol 55, pp 128–140

Exercise Training, Physical Fitness and the Growth Hormone-Insulin-Like Growth Factor-1 Axis and Cytokine Balance

Alon Eliakim · Dan Nemet

Child Health and Sports Center, Endocrinology Clinic, Pediatric Department, Meir Medical Center, Sackler School of Medicine, Tel-Aviv University, Kfar-Saba, Israel

Abstract

The effect of exercise training on anabolic hormones and inflammatory mediators is particularly important during childhood and puberty, since during this period there is a spontaneous increase in anabolic hormones that leads to the marked puberty-related growth spurt. Therefore, any training-associated hormonal and/or inflammatory effect during this critical period may have profound consequences on growth and development, especially if the effect is maintained for long periods. Several studies suggest the hypothesis that a sudden imposition of a training program which is associated with substantial increase in energy expenditure leads initially to an increase in pro-inflammatory cytokines, and as a consequence, to decreases in IGF-1 levels. Further, if the training adaptation is successful, the proinflammatory cytokines fall, and with that decrease, the suppression of IGF-1 diminishes, an anabolic 'rebound' in the GH-IGF-1 axis may ensue, and IGF-1 level exceed the pre-training level. Exactly how and when this switch takes place, and whether the initial catabolic-type stage is necessary for the ultimate anabolic adaptation remains unknown. Consistent with the two phases hypothesis, longer periods of training were indeed associated with stable or with increases in circulating GH and IGF-1 levels. Despite the early training-associated decrease in circulating IGF-1 levels, there is an increase in muscle mass and fitness may improve, suggesting that the local tissue effect of exercise on growth factors differ from systemic effects. Total caloric intake as well as macro-nutrient content, consumption and timing influence the anabolic and inflammatory response to training. Finally, changes in the balance of anabolic and catabolic hormones and inflammatory mediators during the training season may help elite athletes and their coaches in their training and preparation for competition.

Training efficiency depends on the intensity, volume, duration, and frequency of training and on the athlete's ability to tolerate it. An imbalance between the training load and the individual's tolerance may lead to under- or overtraining. As a consequence, many efforts are made to objectively quantify the fine balance between training load and the athlete's tolerance. The endocrine system, by modulation of anabolic and catabolic processes, plays a major role in the physiological adaptation to exercise training [50]. For example, the change in the cortisol/testosterone ratio, as an indicator of the anabolic-catabolic balance, has been used with limited success to determine the physiological strain of training [18]. In recent years changes in circulating components of the growth hormone (GH) → insulin-like growth factor-1 (IGF-1) axis, a system of growth mediators that control somatic and tissue growth in many species [27], have been used to quantify the effects of training [14]. In addition, exercise is also associated with a remarkable change of inflammatory cytokines. These cytokines include both pro-inflammatory mediators [e.g. interleukin-1 (IL-1), IL-6, tumor necrosis factor-α (TNF- α)] and anti-inflammatory mediators [e.g. interleukin-1 receptor antagonist (IL-1ra)] and their response to exercise can be used to gauge exercise load as well. As demonstrated in the previous chapter, the effect of single exercise on these systems is relatively well studied. Surprisingly, single exercise may lead to a simultaneous increase in antagonistic mediators. On the one hand, exercise stimulates anabolic components of the GH → IGF-1 axis [43, 46], while on the other hand, exercise increases catabolic pro-inflammatory cytokines such as IL-6, IL-1 and TNF-α [29, 34, 36]. The assessment of changes in these antagonistic circulating mediators may assist in quantifying the effects of different types of prolonged exercise training and recovery modalities. However, interestingly, relatively few studies examined the levels of these anabolic/catabolic hormones in elite athletes, during different training stages throughout the competitive season, in 'a real life' setting.

The effect of exercise training on these anabolic hormones and inflammatory mediators is particularly important during childhood and puberty, since during this period there is a spontaneous increase in anabolic hormones that leads to the marked puberty-related growth spurt. Therefore, any training-associated hormonal and/or inflammatory effect during this critical period may have profound consequences on growth and development, especially if the effect is maintained for long periods. This chapter will focus on the effect of exercise training on the GH-IGF-1 axis and inflammatory mediators during puberty, on differences between systemic and local (i.e. muscle) responses to exercise and on ways to use these responses to assist adolescent competitive athletes and their coaches in the evaluation of the training load.

Cross-Sectional Relationship between Fitness, Anabolic Hormones and Inflammatory Mediators

Previous studies described [10, 16] that both functional (i.e. maximal oxygen consumption, $\dot{V}O_{2max}$) and structural (i.e. thigh muscle volume determined by magnetic resonance images) indices of fitness were correlated with mean overnight GH levels, GH binding protein (GHBP) and serum IGF-1 levels in pre and late pubertal girls. These cross-sectional data suggest that fitness in healthy, non-professional, pre-pubertal and adolescent females is associated with anabolic adaptations of the GH-IGF-1 system. A recent study in young adult athletes demonstrated that mean and peak GH levels were significantly higher in elite male and female athletes compared to physically active and to sedentary controls with no difference in IGF-1 levels. There was a strong correlation between GH levels and training intensity [49]. Whether the difference in the relationship between fitness and IGF level can be attributed to maturational effect, needs to be elucidated.

The significant correlation between fitness and mean overnight GH levels probably resulted from an increase in peak GH amplitude since only peak amplitude (and not peak frequency or width) correlated with mean GH. The positive correlation between GHBP and fitness is unique. GHBP is the extracellular domain of the GH receptor [41], and therefore reflect tissue GH receptor capacity. Ligand-mediated receptor regulation appears to exist for GH and GHBP in a number of situations. GHBP decreases in acromegaly [24] and during exogenous rhGH therapy [26], and is high in obesity despite low GH [21]. But ligand-mediated receptor downregulation does not appear to operate during normal growth when both GH and GHBP increase in the prepubertal years [4]. The relatively trained or fit state in prepubertal and adolescent females is another example of simultaneous increases in both GH and GHBP. The mechanism of these responses is not known, but suggests anabolic adaptations of both the ligand and receptor. Collectively, it seems that increasing levels of physical activity stimulate GH pulsatility, and, as a consequence, circulating IGF-1. It is compelling to speculate that the stimulation of the GH → IGF-1 axis by exercise contributes, along with genetic, nutritional, and other environmental factors, to an increase in muscle mass and, ultimately, to improved cardiorespiratory responses to exercise (such as peak $\dot{V}O_2$). The data suggest that this mechanism is active both in prepubertal and adolescent girls even while spontaneous growth and natural increase in muscle mass proceeds.

Other studies in adolescent rhythmic gymnasts demonstrated no difference in circulating IGF-1 levels compared to sedentary controls despite reduced adiposity and leptin levels [6]. Since IGF-1 is affected by energy balance, reduced body weight and fat mass is often associated with decreased IGF-1 levels. Therefore, the authors suggested that exercise preserved IGF-1 levels in the rhythmic gymnasts. Consistent with these observations, a follow-up of 4 years during puberty demonstrated that while rhythmic gymnastics training was associated with delayed puberty, there was no effect on linear growth [1].

In contrast, decreased levels of salivary free IGF-1 were found in young female volleyball players compared to sedentary controls [2]. The authors suggested that this decrease could be related to greater muscle requirements. However, whether these results reflect possible different unique body compartment exercise-associated effects (muscle, circulation, saliva) needs to be evaluated.

Virtually all of the major IGF-binding proteins (1 through 6), each of which is known to influence IGF-1 bioactivity in different ways, were also related to indexes of fitness suggesting that the BPs may play a role in the interaction between fitness and exercise. With the exception of IGFBP-3, the level of IGFBPs in the circulation is low, and the exact role of these IGFBPs in the circulation has yet to be determined. Nonetheless, it is noteworthy that the cross-sectional relationships between fitness and IGFBPs were consistent with current understanding of the biological activity of IGF-1-binding proteins based on tissue studies. IGFBP-1 and IGFBP-2, known to inhibit IGF-1 function, were found to be inversely correlated with muscle mass [10, 16]. IGFBP-4, a known inhibitor of the anabolic functions of IGF-1 in bone tissue culture experiments [31], was found to be inversely correlated with muscle mass [10] and $\dot{V}O_{2max}$ [9]. In contrast, the IGF-1 potentiating binding protein, IGFBP-5, was positively correlated with muscle mass [15]. Accordingly, these data suggest the possibility that the generally increased IGF-1 bioactivity in fitter subjects might not be related only to changes in circulating IGF-1, but also to changes in IGFBPs.

Effect of Training

Very few longitudinal studies examined the effect of endurance training on the GH-IGF-1 axis in children. Reduced IGF-1 associated with training has been observed in high school wrestlers and in highly trained young female gymnasts [20, 40]. In these studies, the training program was accompanied by a loss of body mass providing clear evidence for a negative energy balance and catabolic state.

Recently, the effect of a brief (5 weeks) randomized, prospective endurance-type training intervention on the GH-IGF-1 axis in pre and late pubertal males and females was reported. Based on the cross-sectional data, the authors hypothesized that training would lead to increases in circulating GH and IGF-1 levels. Training was accompanied by about 15% higher total energy expenditure (by the doubly labeled water technique), and resulted in significant increases in $\dot{V}O_{2max}$ and thigh muscle volume in the trained but not the control subjects [10, 11, 16, 42]. In contrast to our hypotheses, there was a significant decrease in GHBP, IGF-1 and IGFBP-3 in the trained but not the control prepubertal females [16]; a significant decrease in IGF-1 and IGFBP-3, with a significant increase in IGFBP-2 in the trained but not the control pre-pubertal males [42]; a significant decrease in IGF-1 and IGFBP-5 in the trained but not the control late pubertal females [10], and a significant decrease in GHBP and IGF-1, with a significant increase in IGFBP-2 in the trained, but not control, late pubertal males [11]. Interestingly, endurance training had no effect on GH pulsatility patterns in any of these groups. These effects are commonly observed in energy-deficient states like food deprivation or disease-associated malnutrition [44, 48], but 'catabolic' neuroendocrine adjustments occurred in the present study even though training led to increased thigh muscle volume and was not accompanied by weight loss.

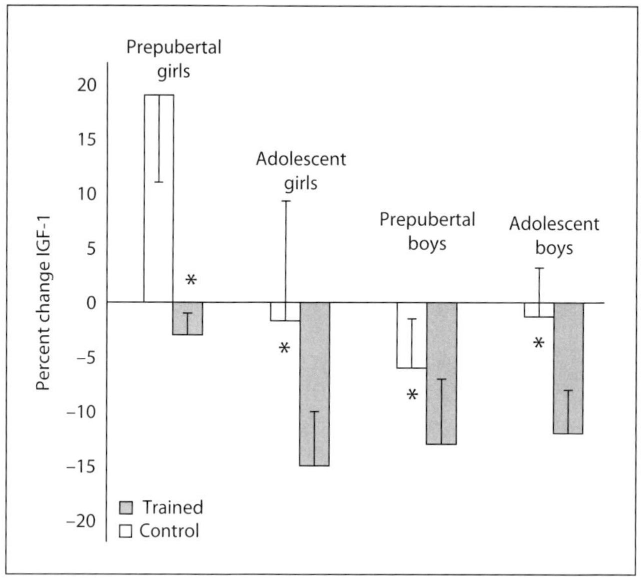

Fig. 1. Effect of a short (5 weeks) endurance-type exercise training on circulating IGF-1 levels in prepubertal and adolescent boys and girls. Training was associated with a significant decrease or attenuated IGF-1 response in all groups.

Thus, the reduction in IGF-1 is sensitive to negative energy balance, but even when energy balance is maintained, exercise training by itself, may lead to small, yet significant reductions in IGF-1 level even in weight-stable subjects [33].

A potential mechanism for this seemingly unexpected systemic 'catabolic-type' adaptation was the reduction in circulating GHBP in the trained subjects. As noted earlier, lower GHBP circulating levels may reflect fewer tissue receptors and reduced tissue responsiveness to GH [41]. As a consequence, since circulating IGF-1 depend on GH-induced hepatic production, IGF-1 levels in the training group decreased. The training effect on GHBP appears to be unique. In several pathological states (malnutrition [38], obesity [21]), the relationship between GH and GHBP suggest the well-described phenomenon of ligand-induced receptor regulation. In this study, training did lead to a reduction in GHBP, but without any change in mean GH or GH pulsatility. Thus, the possibility exists that lower GH receptor is the initiating mechanism in the growth axis response to training. The mechanism for such a direct, training effect on GH receptors or GHBPs is not known.

Interestingly, training was associated with increases in IGFBP-2, a known inhibitor of IGF-1 action, and with reduction in IGFBP-5 in adolescent females. IGFBP-5 is one of the binding proteins that enhance some of the IGF-1 mitogenic effects (i.e. in bones [31]). These observations emphasize again that the exercise training induced decrease in IGF-1 bioavailability is mediated not only by acting on IGF-1 itself, but by altering its binding proteins.

Scheett et al. [42] suggested intriguingly the hypothesis that pro-inflammatory cytokines were involved in the training-induced decreases of IGF-1 (fig. 1). They demonstrated that in a brief 5 weeks' endurance training in prepubertal boys increases in $\dot{V}O_{2max}$ were positively correlated with changes in TNF-α. This suggested that children who trained the hardest and had the biggest increase in fitness also had the largest increase in circulating level of pro-inflammatory cytokines. In addition, changes in IGFBP-3 were inversely correlated with changes in TNF-α and IL-6, suggesting that increase in the inflammatory response mediates the training-associated decrease of components of the GH-IGF-1 axis.

These observations suggest the hypothesis that a sudden imposition of a training program which is associated with substantial increase in energy expenditure leads initially to an increase in pro-inflammatory cytokines, and as a consequence, to decreases in IGF-1 levels. Further, if the training adaptation is successful, the proinflammatory cytokines fall, and with that decrease, the suppression of IGF-1 diminishes, an anabolic 'rebound' in the GH-IGF-1 axis may ensue, and IGF-1 level exceed the pretraining level. Exactly how and when this switch takes place, and whether the initial catabolic-type stage is necessary for the ultimate anabolic adaptation remains unknown.

Adaptations to the training-induced increase in proinflammatory cytokines, and decrease in circulating IGF-1 starts early with training-associated increase in IGF-1 receptor binding capacity [25]. This increase in IGF-1 affinity probably reflects the phenomenon of ligand-mediated receptor upregulation.

Fitter subjects were found to have lower levels of interleukin-1 receptor antagonist (IL-1ra). This agent is stimulated by the inflammatory cytokines and acts to block their biological activity at the receptor level. Therefore, training-associated reduced inflammatory response leads to lower level cytokines and lower steady-state level of IL-1ra. Finally, and consistent with the two phases hypothesis, longer periods of training (5 months [23]), 1 year [51], and 18 months [7] were indeed associated with stable or with increases in circulating GH and IGF-1 levels.

The training-induced increase in muscle mass despite circulating decrease in IGF-1 level suggested that the local tissue effect of exercise on growth factors differ from systemic effects. Very few studies examined the effect of brief exercise or training on skeletal muscle IGF-1 levels. Yan et al. [53] demonstrated that an acute bout of eccentric exercise led to an increase in IGF-1 immunoreactivity in rat type II muscle 4 days postexercise. Consistent with Yan's observation we found [12] that 5 days of treadmill training in young female rats resulted in a significant increase in muscle size and muscle IGF-1 protein, without changes in IGF-1 mRNA, and circulating IGF-1. These results suggest that the early mechanisms of the training adaptation involve translational or posttranslational increases in muscle tissue IGF-1, and that local muscle IGF-1 regulation may be dissociated from central control mechanisms. Along these lines, it was suggested that increases in local IGF-1 was not due to increase in local synthesis, but rather to an increase in IGF-1 uptake from the circulation by a non-membrane-associated IGFBP-1 [37]. This observation emphasizes the possible role of local IGFBPs (which are strongly attached to the cell surface by a

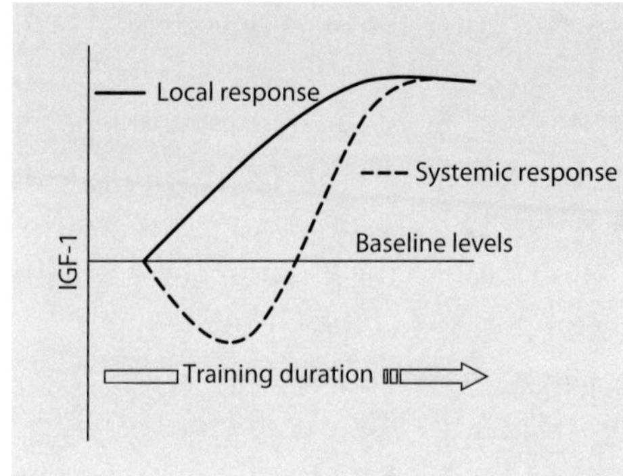

Fig. 2. Differences between local and systemic adaptations of IGF-1 to exercise training. While muscle IGF-1 increases from very early stages of training, there are at least two phases in the systemic IGF-1 response. The first phase is an acute catabolic-type response characterized by a decrease in circulating IGF-1, followed by an anabolic rebound and an increase in IGF-1 levels.

membrane integrin-binding domain) in the regulation of the early adaptation of local IGF-1 to exercise training.

Nevertheless, compensatory hypertrophy of the plantaris and soleus muscle after unilateral excision of the gastrocnemius tendon was accompanied by a significant increase in IGF-1 mRNA after only 2 days (levels of IGF-1 protein were not measured in these study) [8]. This suggests that different types and amount of muscular work could lead to a different time course and pattern of local IGF-1 increase.

Longer periods of exercise training do, however, lead to stimulation of IGF-I gene expression. Zanconato et al. [54] found an increase in hepatic IGF-1 gene expression following 4 weeks of endurance training in young rats. In addition, the authors showed that the 4 weeks of endurance type training led to increases in the exercising muscle IGF-1 gene expression and protein. Interestingly, inhibition of GH (by hypophysectomy [8] or by GH-releasing hormone antibody [54]) actually enhanced the local IGF-1 response to increased muscular effort. It is clear from these observations that inhibition of GH alone cannot block the autocrine and paracrine effects of IGF-1, emphasizing the GH independence of the 'local' IGF-1 anabolic adaptations to physical activity.

What is the advantage of simultaneous central catabolism and local anabolism early in the adaptation to increased physical activity? This adaptive mechanism might reduce global anabolic function thereby conserving energy sources, but still allow for local tissue growth in response to environmental stresses like exercise training (fig. 2).

Consistent with this speculation is the phenomenon of attenuated somatic growth and reduced circulating IGF-1 despite muscle adaptation to intense exercise training in nutritionally, self-deprived young elite athletes (e.g. female gymnasts [47]). The dissociation between target tissue and circulating GH-IGF-1 responses was demonstrated also in other environmental conditions [32]. Rats exposed to hypoxia had reduced growth rate and circulating IGF-1, but, their heart and lung size, along with local IGF-1 gene expression, was increased. This indicates that local anabolic adjustment to reduced oxygen carrying capacity had occurred, but the central response was catabolic and overall growth was reduced.

The Young Competitive Athlete – Useful Applications

Measurements of IGF-1 levels can also assist the athlete and coach in the preparation for competition. The effect of 4 weeks of training on fitness, self-assessment physical conditioning scores and circulating IGF-1 was previously determined [13] in elite professional handball players during their preparation for the junior world championships. Training consisted of 2 weeks of intense training followed by 2 weeks of relative tapering. Circulating IGF-1 and physical conditioning scores decreased initially, and returned to baseline levels at the end of training. There was a significant positive correlation between the changes in circulating IGF-1 and the physical conditioning scores suggesting that the athlete's self-assessment might serve as a reliable tool when laboratory assistance is unavailable. Consistent with these findings, a follow-up of IGF-1 levels during the training season in elite adolescent wrestlers showed also a decrease in IGF-1 level during periods of heavy training, and return to baseline during tapering down and prior to the competition season [35]. Interestingly, changes in the pro- and anti-inflammatory mediators IL-6 and IL-1ra correlated negatively with changes in IGF-1, being high when IGF-1 level were low, and normalized when IGF-1 levels normalized, emphasizing their potential contributing role for the training-associated change in IGF-1 (fig. 3). Similarly, levels of IGF-1 and the ratio of IGF-1/BP-3 as an index of the bioactive free IGF-1 increased significantly throughout the competitive season in late pubertal triathletes [28].

Tapering down the training intensity prior to the competition is a well-known training methodology to help the athlete to achieve his best performance [45]. This strategy is indeed associated with a parallel increase in circulating IGF-1 levels. Therefore, these measures may assist coaches and athletes in their training preparations. Interestingly, in type of sports that do not plan their training for a specific target, and train in the relative same intensity throughout the season (e.g. soccer), changes in IGF-1 level and its major binding protein IGFBP-3, were not found [30].

In optimal conditions, during the tapering of training intensity, IGF-1 level will increase above baseline levels and will be associated with improved performance, however, this does not occur always. Since IGF-1 can be reduced by weight loss, it is possible that a deliberate decrease in body weight in athletes who participate in weight category sports (e.g. judokas, wrestlers) prior to major championships may prevent further increase in this anabolic hormone, and will be associated 'only' with a significant return to baseline values [35, 40]. Moreover, previous studies demonstrated training-associated negative correlation between circulating IGF-1 and ghrelin, a hormone that is secreted by the stomach and pancreas and known to stimulate hunger, in athletes [22]. These hormonal relationships can play a role in the training-induced changes in energy balance and body composition, in particularly in weight category sports.

As noted earlier, despite the decrease in circulating IGF-1 [10, 11, 16, 42] during a period of intense training, fitness may still improve. This suggests that while

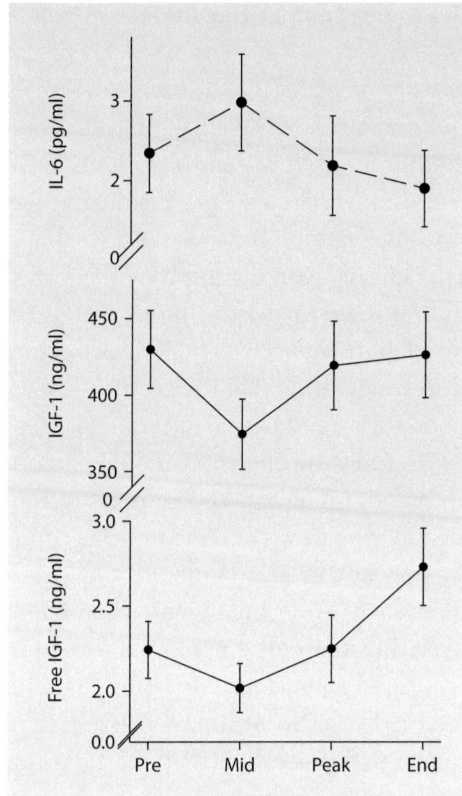

Fig. 3. The effect of a wrestling season on IL-6, total and free IGF-1 circulating levels. Following an initial decrease, total IGF-1 levels returned to baseline at end season while free IGF-1 rebounded reaching an above baseline levels. IL-6 followed an inverse pattern.

changes in circulating IGF-1 are good markers of the general condition and energy balance of the athlete, they are not necessarily good predictors of the athlete's performance. Probably, it is the local muscle levels of these hormones, and their autocrine or paracrine secretion, that is more indicative of skeletal muscle performance [17, 54]. Tapering of the training intensity, however, was found to be associated with both increased IGF-1 level and with improvement of exercise performance of the athletes [19, 45].

It is still unknown what should be the permitted decrease of IGF-1 levels during periods of heavy training, or what should be the optimal increase of this substance during periods of tapering down and reduced training intensity. However, we believe that an inability to increase circulating IGF-1 levels before the target competition should be an alarming sign for both the athlete and his/her coach that the athlete's general condition is not optimal. Collection of baseline and training-related hormonal changes, with a comparison to the hormonal response in previous seasons, and the knowledge and experience of the past success may prove to be of a very significant relevance as well.

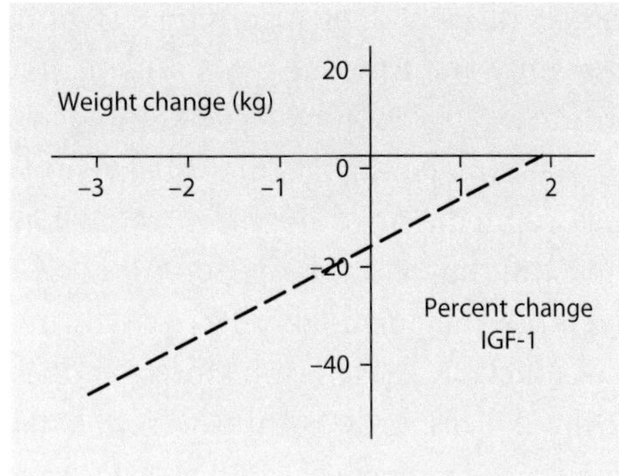

Fig. 4. Changes in IGF-1 associated with exercise training as a function of percent change in body weight. A decrease following training was observed even when weight was unchanged.

Exercise, Nutrition and the Growth Axis

It was suggested that the main cause for the initial decrease in anabolic components of the GH-IGF-1 axis in pubertal athletes is nutritional deficit. A recent report examined the effect of caloric restriction compared to caloric supplementation (calculated to maintain positive energy balance) during 7 days of heavy training (3 h/day) in late adolescent wrestlers. The study demonstrated that while negative energy balance was associated with IGF-1 decrease, adequate nutrition attenuated the decrease in IGF-1 levels. However, it was demonstrated that a small decrease in IGF-1 level may occur even when energy balance and weight stability were maintained [33] (fig. 4). Moreover, wrestlers in the caloric supplemented group stated that it was very hard to follow the dietary guidelines, suggesting that the optimal conditions of feeding might not exist in 'real life' training situation.

Several studies suggested that the timing of nutritional supplementation may affect the training-associated response of the GH-IGF-1 axis. Protein supplementation one hour prior and after practice during 10 weeks of resistance training (4 times/week) were more effective than carbohydrate placebo in increasing muscle mass and muscle strength and were associated with greater increases in IGF-1 and IGF-1 mRNA in untrained males [52]. Consistent with these findings, twice daily protein compared to carbohydrate supplementation during 6 months of strength and conditioning training (5 times/week) was associated with greater increase in IGF-1 levels in untrained late pubertal and young adult males and females [3]. Bovine colostrums supplementation during 8 weeks of resistance and plyometric training resulted in a significant increase in anaerobic power, but had no effect on alactic anaerobic capacity or plasma IGF-I levels [5]. In contrast, Rankin et al. [39] studied the effect of immediate postexercise milk compared to carbohydrate-electrolyte drink consumption during 10 weeks of resistance training in untrained late pubertal and young adults and found no difference in body composition, muscle strength and IGF-1 level changes. These results suggest that macronutrient content and consumption, and not only the total caloric intake, influence the GH-IGF-1 response to training. This information is particularly important for the child athlete, mainly during period of maturation and rapid growth.

In summary, changes in the balance of anabolic and catabolic hormones and inflammatory mediators during the training season may help elite athletes and coaches in their training and preparation for competition. Further studies are needed, however, to clarify the hormonal response during different phases of training to enable optimal athletic achievement. Moreover, the complex relationship of the exercise induced hormonal response with nutritional status and pre- and postexercise supplementation during periods of rapid growth warrants further research.

References

1 Adiyaman P, Ocal G, Berberoglu M, Evliyaoglu O, Aycan Z, Cetinkaya E, Bulca Y, Ersoz G, Akar N: Alterations in serum growth hormone (GH)/GH dependent ternary complex components (IGF-I, IGFBP-3, ALS, IGF-I/IGFBP-3 molar ratio) and the influence of these alterations on growth pattern in female rhythmic gymnasts. J Pediatr Endocrinol Metab 2004;17:895–903.

2 Antonelli G, Cappellin E, Gatti R, Chiappin S, Spinella P, De Palo EF: Measurement of free IGF-I saliva levels: perspectives in the detection of GH/IGF axis in athletes. Clin Biochem 2007;40:545–550.

3 Ballard TL, Clapper JA, Specker BL, Binkley TL, Vukovich MD: Effect of protein supplementation during a 6-mo strength and conditioning program on insulin-like growth factor I and markers of bone turnover in young adults. Am J Clin Nutr 2005;81:1442–1448.

4 Baumann G, Shaw MA, Amburn K: Regulation of plasma growth hormone-binding proteins in health and disease. Metabolism 1989;38:683–689.

5 Buckley JD, Brinkworth GD, Abbott MJ: Effect of bovine colostrum on anaerobic exercise performance and plasma insulin-like growth factor I. J Sports Sci 2003;21:577–588.

6 Courteix D, Rieth N, Thomas T, Van PE, Benhamou CL, Collomp K, Lespessailles E, Jaffre C: Preserved bone health in adolescent elite rhythmic gymnasts despite hypoleptinemia. Horm Res 2007;68:20–27.

7 Daly RM, Rich PA, Klein R, Bass S: Effects of high-impact exercise on ultrasonic and biochemical indices of skeletal status: a prospective study in young male gymnasts. J Bone Miner Res 1999;14:1222–1230.

8 DeVol DL, Rotwein P, Sadow JL, Novakofski J, Bechtel PJ: Activation of insulin-like growth factor gene expression during work-induced skeletal muscle growth. Am J Physiol 1990;259:E89–E95.

9 Eliakim A, Brasel JA, Barstow TJ, Mohan S, Cooper DM: Peak oxygen uptake, muscle volume, and the growth hormone-insulin-like growth factor-I axis in adolescent males. Med Sci Sports Exerc 1998;30:512–517.

10 Eliakim A, Brasel JA, Mohan S, Barstow TJ, Berman N, Cooper DM: Physical fitness, endurance training, and the growth hormone-insulin-like growth factor I system in adolescent females. J Clin Endocrinol Metab 1996;81:3986–3992.

11 Eliakim A, Brasel JA, Mohan S, Wong WL, Cooper DM: Increased physical activity and the growth hormone-IGF-I axis in adolescent males. Am J Physiol 1998;275:R308–R314.

12 Eliakim A, Moromisato M, Moromisato D, Brasel JA, Roberts C Jr, Cooper DM: Increase in muscle IGF-I protein but not IGF-I mRNA after 5 days of endurance training in young rats. Am J Physiol 1997;273:R1557–R1561.

13 Eliakim A, Nemet D, Bar-Sela S, Higer Y, Falk B: Changes in circulating IGF-I and their correlation with self-assessment and fitness among elite athletes. Int J Sports Med 2002;23:600–603.

14 Eliakim A, Nemet D, Cooper DM: Exercise, training and the GH->IGF-I axis; in Kraemer WJ, Rogol A.D (eds): The Endocrine System in Sports and Exercise. Oxford, Wiley-Blackwell, 2005, vol 11, pp 165–179.

15 Eliakim A, Scheett T, Allmendinger N, Brasel JA, Cooper DM: Training, muscle volume, and energy expenditure in nonobese American girls. J Appl Physiol 2001;90:35–44.

16 Eliakim A, Scheett TP, Newcomb R, Mohan S, Cooper DM: Fitness, training, and the growth hormone->insulin-like growth factor I axis in prepubertal girls. J Clin Endocrinol Metab 2001;86:2797–2802.

17 Greig CA, Hameed M, Young A, Goldspink G, Noble B: Skeletal muscle IGF-I isoform expression in healthy women after isometric exercise. Growth Horm IGF Res 2006;16:373–376.
18 Hoffman JR, Falk B, Radom-Isaac S, Weinstein Y, Magazanik A, Wang Y, Yarom Y: The effect of environmental temperature on testosterone and cortisol responses to high intensity, intermittent exercise in humans. Eur J Appl Physiol Occup Physiol 1997;75:83–87.
19 Izquierdo M, Ibanez J, Gonzalez-Badillo JJ, Ratamess NA, Kraemer WJ, Hakkinen K, Bonnabau H, Granados C, French DN, Gorostiaga EM: Detraining and tapering effects on hormonal responses and strength performance. J Strength Cond Res 2007;21:768–775.
20 Jahreis G, Kauf E, Frohner G, Schmidt HE: Influence of intensive exercise on insulin-like growth factor I, thyroid and steroid hormones in female gymnasts. Growth Regul 1991;1:95–99.
21 Jorgensen JO, Pedersen SB, Borglum J, Frystyk J, Ho KK, Christiansen JS, Orskov H, Blum WF, Richelsen B: Serum concentrations of insulin-like growth factors (IGFs), IGF binding proteins 1 and 3 and growth hormone binding protein in obese women and the effects of growth hormone administration: a double-blind, placebo-controlled study. Eur J Endocrinol 1995;133:65–70.
22 Jurimae J, Cicchella A, Jurimae T, Latt E, Haljaste K, Purge P, Hamra J, von Duvillard SP: Regular physical activity influences plasma ghrelin concentration in adolescent girls. Med Sci Sports Exerc 2007;39:1736–1741.
23 Koziris LP, Hickson RC, Chatterton RT Jr, Groseth RT, Christie JM, Goldflies DG, Unterman TG: Serum levels of total and free IGF-I and IGFBP-3 are increased and maintained in long-term training. J Appl Physiol 1999;86:1436–1442.
24 Kratzsch J, Blum WF, Ventz M, Selisko T, Birkenmeyer G, Keller E: Growth hormone-binding protein-related immunoreactivity in the serum of patients with acromegaly is regulated inversely by growth hormone concentration. Eur J Endocrinol 1995;132:306–312.
25 Lee C, Eliakim A, Brasel JA, Cooper DM: Effect of exercise training on erythrocyte insulin-like growth factor-I receptor binding in adolescent males. J Pediatr Endocrinol Metab 2000;13:621–627.
26 Leger J, Noel M, Czernichow P, Postel-Vinay MC: Progressive normalization of growth hormone-binding protein and IGF-I levels in treated growth hormone-deficient children. Pediatr Res 1995;37:731–735.
27 LeRoith D, Roberts CT Jr: Insulin-like growth factors and their receptors in normal physiology and pathological states. J Pediatr Endocrinol 1993;6:251–255.
28 Maimoun L, Galy O, Manetta J, Coste O, Peruchon E, Micallef JP, Mariano-Goulart D, Couret I, Sultan C, Rossi M: Competitive season of triathlon does not alter bone metabolism and bone mineral status in male triathletes. Int J Sports Med 2004;25:230–234.
29 Meckel Y, Eliakim A, Seraev M, Zaldivar F, Cooper DM, Sagiv M, Nemet D: The effect of a brief sprint interval exercise on growth factors and inflammatory mediators. J Strength Cond Res 2009;23:225–230.
30 Mejri S, Bchir F, Ben Rayana MC, Ben HJ, Ben SC: Effect of training on GH and IGF-1 responses to a submaximal exercise in football players. Eur J Appl Physiol 2005;95:496–503.
31 Mohan S, Nakao Y, Honda Y, Landale E, Leser U, Dony C, Lang K, Baylink DJ: Studies on the mechanisms by which insulin-like growth factor (IGF) binding protein-4 (IGFBP-4) and IGFBP-5 modulate IGF actions in bone cells. J Biol Chem 1995;270:20424–20431.
32 Moromisato DY, Moromisato MY, Brasel JA, Cooper DM: Effect of growth hormone therapy in mitigating hypoxia-induced and food restriction-induced growth retardation in the newborn rat. Crit Care Med 1999;27:2234–2238.
33 Nemet D, Connolly PH, Pontello-Pescatello AM, Rose-Gottron C, Larson JK, Galassetti P, Cooper DM: Negative energy balance plays a major role in the IGF-I response to exercise training. J Appl Physiol 2004;96:276–282.
34 Nemet D, Oh Y, Kim HS, Hill M, Cooper DM: Effect of intense exercise on inflammatory cytokines and growth mediators in adolescent boys. Pediatrics 2002;110:681–689.
35 Nemet D, Pontello AM, Rose-Gottron C, Cooper DM: Cytokines and growth factors during and after a wrestling season in adolescent boys. Med Sci Sports Exerc 2004;36:794–800.
36 Nemet D, Rose-Gottron CM, Mills PJ, Cooper DM: Effect of water polo practice on cytokines, growth mediators, and leukocytes in girls. Med Sci Sports Exerc 2003;35:356–363.
37 Phillip M, Werner H, Palese T, Kowarski AA, Stannard B, Bach LA, LeRoith D, Roberts CT Jr: Differential accumulation of insulin-like growth factor-I in kidneys of pre- and postpubertal streptozotocin-diabetic rats. J Mol Endocrinol 1994;12:215–224.
38 Postel-Vinay MC, Saab C, Gourmelen M: Nutritional status and growth hormone-binding protein. Horm Res 1995;44:177–181.
39 Rankin JW, Goldman LP, Puglisi MJ, Nickols-Richardson SM, Earthman CP, Gwazdauskas FC: Effect of post-exercise supplement consumption on adaptations to resistance training. J Am Coll Nutr 2004;23:322–330.

40 Roemmich JN, Sinning WE: Weight loss and wrestling training: effects on growth-related hormones. J Appl Physiol 1997;82:1760–1764.

41 Rosenfeld RG: Circulating growth hormone binding proteins. Horm Res 1994;42:129–132.

42 Scheett TP, Nemet D, Stoppani J, Maresh CM, Newcomb R, Cooper DM: The effect of endurance-type exercise training on growth mediators and inflammatory cytokines in pre-pubertal and early pubertal males. Pediatr Res 2002;52:491–497.

43 Schwarz AJ, Brasel JA, Hintz RL, Mohan S, Cooper DM: Acute effect of brief low- and high-intensity exercise on circulating insulin-like growth factor (IGF) I, II, and IGF-binding protein-3 and its proteolysis in young healthy men. J Clin Endocrinol Metab 1996;81:3492–3497.

44 Smith WJ, Underwood LE, Clemmons DR: Effects of caloric or protein restriction on insulin-like growth factor-I (IGF-I) and IGF-binding proteins in children and adults. J Clin Endocrinol Metab 1995;80:443–449.

45 Steinacker JM, Lormes W, Kellmann M, Liu Y, Reissnecker S, Opitz-Gress A, Baller B, Gunther K, Petersen KG, Kallus KW, Lehmann M, Altenburg D: Training of junior rowers before world championships: effects on performance, mood state and selected hormonal and metabolic responses. J Sports Med Phys Fitness 2000;40:327–335.

46 Stokes K, Nevill M, Frystyk J, Lakomy H, Hall G: Human growth hormone responses to repeated bouts of sprint exercise with different recovery periods between bouts 3. J Appl Physiol 2005;99:1254–1261.

47 Theintz GE, Howald H, Weiss U, Sizonenko PC: Evidence for a reduction of growth potential in adolescent female gymnasts. J Pediatr 1993;122:306–313.

48 Tonshoff B, Blum WF, Wingen AM, Mehls O: Serum insulin-like growth factors (IGFs) and IGF binding proteins 1, 2, and 3 in children with chronic renal failure: relationship to height and glomerular filtration rate. The European Study Group for Nutritional Treatment of Chronic Renal Failure in Childhood. J Clin Endocrinol Metab 1995;80:2684–2691.

49 Ubertini G, Grossi A, Colabianchi D, Fiori R, Brufani C, Bizzarri C, Giannone G, Rigamonti AE, Sartorio A, Muller EE, Cappa M: Young elite athletes of different sport disciplines present with an increase in pulsatile secretion of growth hormone compared with non-elite athletes and sedentary subjects. J Endocrinol Invest 2008;31:138–145.

50 Urhausen A, Kindermann W: The endocrine system in overtraining; in Warren MP, Constantini NW (eds): Sports Endocrinology. New Jersey, Humana Press, 2000 pp 347–370.

51 Weltman A, Weltman JY, Schurrer R, Evans WS, Veldhuis JD, Rogol AD: Endurance training amplifies the pulsatile release of growth hormone: effects of training intensity. J Appl Physiol 1992;72:2188–2196.

52 Willoughby DS, Stout JR, Wilborn CD: Effects of resistance training and protein plus amino acid supplementation on muscle anabolism, mass, and strength. Amino Acids 2007;32:467–477.

53 Yan Z, Biggs RB, Booth FW: Insulin-like growth factor immunoreactivity increases in muscle after acute eccentric contractions. J Appl Physiol 1993;74:410–414.

54 Zanconato S, Moromisato DY, Moromisato MY, Woods J, Brasel JA, LeRoith D, Roberts CT Jr, Cooper DM: Effect of training and growth hormone suppression on insulin-like growth factor I mRNA in young rats. J Appl Physiol 1994;76:2204–2209.

Alon Eliakim, MD
Department of Pediatrics, Child Health and Sports Center
Meir Medical Center
Kfar-Saba, 44281 (Israel)
Tel. +972 9 7472134, Fax +972 9 7471303, E-Mail Eliakim.alon@clalit.org.il

Jürimäe J, Hills AP, Jürimäe T (eds): Cytokines, Growth Mediators and Physical Activity in Children during Puberty.
Med Sport Sci. Basel, Karger, 2010, vol 55, pp 141–155

Growth Hormone-Insulin-Like Growth Factor-1 and Inflammatory Response to a Single Exercise Bout in Children and Adolescents

Dan Nemet · Alon Eliakim

Child Health and Sports Center, Endocrinology clinic, Pediatric Department, Meir Medical Center, Sackler School of Medicine, Tel-Aviv University, Kfar-Saba, Israel

Abstract

Physical activity plays an important role in tissue anabolism, growth and development, but the mechanisms that link patterns of exercise with tissue anabolism are not completely understood. The effectiveness of physical training depends on the training load and on the individual ability to tolerate it, and an imbalance between the two may lead to under or over-training. Therefore, many efforts have been made to find objective parameters to quantify the balance between training load and the athlete's tolerance. One of the unique features of exercise is that it leads to a simultaneous increase of antagonistic mediators. On the one hand, exercise stimulates anabolic components of the growth hormone (GH) → IGF-1 (insulin-like growth factor-1) axis. On the other hand, exercise elevates catabolic pro-inflammatory cytokines such as interleukin-6 (IL-6), IL-1 and tumor necrosis factor-α (TNF-α). This emphasizes probably the importance of optimal adaptation to exercise in particularly during adolescence. The very fine balance between the anabolic and inflammatory/catabolic response to exercise will determine the effectiveness of exercise training and the health consequences of exercise. If the anabolic response is stronger, exercise will probably lead ultimately to increased muscle mass and improved fitness. A greater catabolic response, in particularly if persists for long duration, may lead to overtraining. Therefore, changes in the anabolic-catabolic hormonal balance and in circulating inflammatory cytokines can be used by adolescent athletes and/or their coaches to gauge the training intensity in individual and team sports.

Physical activity plays an important role in tissue anabolism, growth and development, but the mechanisms that link patterns of exercise with tissue anabolism are not completely understood. The anabolic effects of exercise are not limited to individuals participating in competitive sports since substantial anabolic stimulus arises even from the relatively modest physical activity of daily living [1].

The exercise-associated anabolic effects are age and maturity dependent. Naturally occurring levels of physical activity are significantly higher during childhood, and simultaneously there is a substantial increase in muscle mass and strength during adolescence. Thus, the combination of rapid growth and development, high levels of physical activity and spontaneous puberty-related increases in anabolic hormones (growth hormone [GH], insulin-like growth factor-1 [IGF-1], and sex steroids) suggests the possibility of integrated mechanisms linking exercise with a variety of anabolic responses. On the other hand, participation of young athletes in intense competitive training, especially if associated with inadequate caloric intake, may lead to several health hazards, and may reduce growth potential [2]. It is now well established that the translation of physical activity to health effects rests on the interaction of seemingly dichotomous anabolic and catabolic mediators and cell signaling pathways including growth factors like GH and IGF-1 and inflammatory cytokines like interleukin-6 (IL-6).

This chapter will focus on the effect of a single exercise bout on components of the GH-IGF-1 axis in children and adolescents, and will emphasize the unique relationship between the exercise-related anabolic response and exercise-associated change in inflammatory mediators. In addition, since the participation of children and adolescents in competitive sport is increasing in recent years, we will suggest the possible role of analyzing the GH-IGF-1 and inflammatory response to exercise in order to assist competitive athletes and their coaches in the evaluation of the training load and competition preparation.

GH-IGF-1 Axis

The GH-IGF-1 axis is composed of hormones, growth factors, binding proteins (BP) and receptors that regulate essential life processes such as growth and development, metabolic and reparative processes and aging. Therefore, to understand the axis one must consider each individual component and the interaction between them, under both physiologic and pathological conditions. The axis starts at the level of the central nervous system where several neurotransmitters (catecholamines, serotonin and cholinergic agents, etc.) stimulate the hypothalamus to synthesize growth hormone-releasing hormone (GHRH) and somatostatin (SMS). GHRH stimulates the anterior pituitary to synthesize and secrete GH, while SMS inhibits GH secretion.

GH is the major product of the axis. One of the most important functions of GH is the stimulation of hepatic IGF-I synthesis. However, some effects of GH on metabolism, body composition and tissue differentiation are IGF-1 independent. GH exerts a direct feedback mechanism on the two hypothalamic hormones that control its secretion. Tissue GH bioactivity results from an interaction between GH and the GH receptor and the GH receptor is composed of intracellular and extracellular trans-membrane domains. The extracellular domain is identical in structure to the GH-binding protein (GHBP) [3]; therefore, a unique feature of this axis is that GH receptor number and activity can be determined easily by measurements of circulating GHBP levels.

IGF-1 is one of the insulin-related peptides which can act as a hormone and these effects are GH-dependent. However, the majority of IGF-1's actions occur due to paracrine or autocrine secretion and regulation, which are only partially GH-dependent. IGF-1 is responsible for most, but not all, anabolic and growth related effects of GH. IGF-1 also stimulates SMS secretion, and inhibits GH by a negative feedback mechanism [4]. It is not clear whether this feedback mechanism is caused by circulating or local central IGF-1.

The bulk of circulating IGF-1 is bound to several insulin-like growth factor-binding proteins (IGFBPs). The most important circulating BP is IGFBP-3, which is synthesized mainly in the liver. When bound to IGF-1, the IGBP complexes with an acid-labile subunit to form a circulating ternary complex that carries most of the IGF-1 in the serum. Some IGFBPs are GH dependent (e.g. IGFBP-3), but others, like IGFBP-1 and IGFBP-2, are insulin-dependent (being high when insulin level is low). The interaction between IGF-1 and its BPs is even more complicated since some BPs stimulate (e.g. IGFBP-5), while others inhibit (e.g. IGFBP-4) IGF-1 anabolic effects [5].

The effects of IGF-1 result from its interaction with two different receptors. The type 1 receptor has tyrosine-kinase activity, and mediates most of the IGF-1 effects. This receptor exhibits similarities to the insulin receptor, and therefore may also bind with insulin which has known anabolic effects. The type 2 receptor is identical to the mannose 6-phosphate receptor and binds IGF-2 as well.

Some hormones in the GH-IGF-1 axis (i.e. GHRH, SMS and GH) have a pulsatile secretion pattern, and it has been shown that the pulsatility of GH secretion is significantly important for accelerated growth rate [6]. In contrast, the IGF-1 and IGFBP levels are relatively stable throughout the day. In addition to the important effect on growth, GH and IGF-1 have a marked effect on body composition. Both hormones stimulate increases in muscle mass and bone mineral density, and reduce fat distribution.

Several components of the axis are age-dependent. For example, GHRH, GH, GHBP, IGF-1 and IGFBP-3 all reach their peak circulating levels during puberty [7] and decrease with aging [8]. These changes are partially sex-hormone-mediated; however, nutritional state also has a remarkable influence on the GH-IGF-1 axis. For example, fasting and malnutrition increase GH secretion, but despite elevated GH, IGF-1 levels are reduced due to a lower level of GH receptors [9]. All of these factors must be taken into account when studying the effect of exercise on the GH-IGF-1 axis and its components.

Inflammatory Cytokines

In adults, Ostrowski et al. [10] noted that strenuous exercise stimulated pro-inflammatory mediators, but simultaneously, '...cytokine inhibitors and anti-inflammatory cytokines restrict the magnitude and duration of the inflammatory response to exercise'. Single bouts of exercise in children could, like in adults, stimulate both pro-inflammatory cytokines, known to directly inhibit the anabolic activity of the GH→IGF-1 axis (namely, IL-6, IL-1β, and TNF-α) as well as anti-inflammatory mediators that may promote growth. The balance between these systems will ultimately determine whether exercise would lead to beneficial or detrimental effects [11].

Effect of a Single Exercise Bout

Growth Hormone

The GH response to exercise depends on the duration and intensity of the exercise bout, the fitness level of the exercising individual, the timing of blood sampling, refractoriness of pituitary GH secretion to the exercise stimuli, and other environmental factors. Therefore, standardized exercise protocols should be used in order to properly evaluate the GH response to acute exercise [12].

Our current knowledge on the exercise-associated GH response is mainly related to aerobic-type exercise. While previous reports suggested that less fit individuals exhibit a greater GH response to exercise [13], individuals in these studies performed exercise at the same *absolute,* rather than *relative*, capacity. Since fitness level varied markedly among participants, some participants exercised below, while others exercise above, their lactate/anaerobic threshold (LAT). This is important since it was shown that GH levels increase only in response to endurance exercise intensity above the LAT [14], and that an exercise intensity of 75–90% of the maximal aerobic power yielded greater GH increase than less intense loads [15, 16]. These results simply demonstrate that as individuals become fitter, the stress associated with exercise at an absolute work rate diminishes. This suggests that the same *relative* exercise intensity should preferably be used to study the 'real' GH response. This scientific approach mandates, therefore, evaluation of the maximal oxygen capacity and/or LAT, and calculation of the relative exercise intensity in order to determine the GH response.

Exercise duration for the stimulation of GH secretion should be at least 10 minutes, since a shorter duration (e.g. 5 min at above the LAT] was not accompanied by increased GH levels [14]. The exercise-induced GH peak occurs 25–30 min after the start of the exercise, irrespective of the exercise length [17–20]. In females, the GH peak occurs a few minutes earlier than in males [18]. Moreover, in about 90% of children the GH peak occurs 20–40 min after the start of exercise. Thus, in a brief exercise period (e.g. 10 min), the peak will be reached after the end of exercise, while in a longer duration exercise session (e.g. 60 min), the peak will be reached during exercise period. Blood sampling, in any case, should be timed to the exercise-induced GH peak. Multiple GH sampling (e.g. 20, 30 and 40 min after the start of exercise) will probably prove to be more accurate in determining the 'true' individual GH peak.

While analyzing the GH response to exercise, it is important to consider the pituitary refractoriness, namely, the time in which the normal pituitary gland will not respond sufficiently to exercise stimulation for GH release. We previously demonstrated [21] that the GH response to exercise was inhibited if a spontaneous, early morning, GH pulse had occurred within 1 h prior to the exercise test. This inhibition probably resulted from GH autoinhibition (previously elevated circulating GH attenuated the pituitary's response to exercise). Cappon et al. [22] previously demonstrated at least a 1-hour refractory period following exercise-induced GH secretion (i.e. a subsequent GH response to exercise was blunted), and suggested that an exercise-induced increase in free fatty acids or alterations in parasympathetic/sympathetic tone might have been responsible [22, 23]. Ronsen et al. [24] showed that if the second high intensity endurance exercise bout was performed 3 h after the first session, GH peak did occur. Similarly, integrated 1.5 h GH concentrations were found to be significantly greater if the difference between exercise bouts (30 min, 70% VO_{2max}) was 3.5 h [25]. This indicated that young competitive athletes who practice several times every day should plan for a sufficient interval between multiple daily exercise sessions.

The majority of studies to date have focused on the effect of endurance type exercise on GH secretion, however recently, efforts have been made to characterize the GH response to anaerobic-type exercise. A significant increase in GH levels was found following the Wingate Anaerobic Test (30 s of supramaximal cycle exercise against resistance that is calculated relative to each individual's body mass) in young adults [26]. More recently, we demonstrated a significant increase in GH levels following a typical volleyball practice [27], and following different types of interval training [constant distance: 4 × 250 m; increasing distances: 100–200–300–400 m; decreasing distances: 400–300–200–100 m] [28]. This is important since children's daily physical activity is characterized mainly by spontaneous, short anaerobic-type bouts suggesting that GH response to this kind of exercise may better represent their activities [29].

Both aerobic and anaerobic exercises that stimulated GH secretion involved high metabolic demands. In contrast, we previously demonstrated a smaller but still significant GH response to exercise input that was perceived as difficult by the participants (i.e. 10 min of unilateral wrist flexion; a small and relatively unused muscle group), but had no systemic effect on heart rate or circulating lactate levels [30]. This suggests that other features like an individual's perceived exertion and associated psychological stress may also activate the hypothalamic-pituitary axis and GH release even in exercise involving small muscle groups.

Environmental factors like nutrition may also interfere with the GH response to exercise. For example, intravenous administration of the amino acid arginine is a strong stimulator of GH release and is used as one of the common provocation tests for GH secretion in the assessment of children with short stature. In contrast, the ingestion of a lipid-rich meal 45–60 min prior to an intermittent 30 min cycle-ergometer exercise resulted in a significant, >40% reduction in the GH secretion in healthy children [31]. The effect of prior high-fat meal ingestion appeared to be selective for GH, as other counter-regulatory responses to exercise, such as glucagon, cortisol and epinephrine, were not affected. In adults, the high fat meal related exercise-induced GH secretion inhibition was correlated with circulating somatostatin levels. Interestingly, a high carbohydrate meal with a similar caloric content was associated with a smaller, nonsignificant decrease in GH response to exercise. The effect of a high protein meal on exercise-induced GH secretion in children was not studied. Since the GH response to exercise plays an important role in muscle adaptation to exercise, these studies indicate that adolescent athletes should avoid consumption of high fat meal prior to each practice to ensure optimal GH response.

Exercise-associated GH release is attenuated in amenorrheic athletes, due to decreased GHRH response to exercise compared to eumenorrheic athletes [32–35]. This is particularly relevant to the adolescent female athlete, since the prevalence of amenorrhea among these athletes is 4–20 times higher than the general population. 'Athletic amenorrhea' appears mainly in younger athletes, in sports where leanness can provide a competitive advantage (e.g. aesthetic-type sports, long distance running), and, in particular, when intense training is accompanied by inadequate nutrition [36]. The reduced exercise-induced GH response in these athletes should be considered since it probably indicates reduced training effectiveness.

Pathological conditions like childhood obesity may also affect the GH response to exercise. A significantly reduced exercise-associated GH response was reported in otherwise healthy obese children and adolescents [37]. The GH response of obese individuals was also attenuated following other commonly used agents for GH provocation tests [38]. An attenuated catecholamine response to exercise was also found in obese children. This is important since childhood obesity has now reached epidemic proportions and a prevalence of 20–25% in Westernized societies. It is possible that the blunted GH and catecholamine response to exercise leads to reduced carbohydrate and fat utilization during exercise in obese children [39], and, as a result, to a greater protein utilization. This may, at least partially, explain the difficulties in achieving changes in body composition and an increase muscle mass by exercise interventions in obese children. Consistent with this, previous studies have demonstrated that elevated BMI was associated with a reduced training effect in children following a prolonged resistance training intervention. Therefore, it is possible that the GH and catecholamine response to exercise might be used prior to participation in weight reduction interventions to predict the outcome of these interventions. A sufficient GH and catecholamine response would be predictive of success, whereas an insufficient response would indicate a need for a more intense intervention. Further studies are needed to clarify the extent to which these hormonal abnormalities persist after

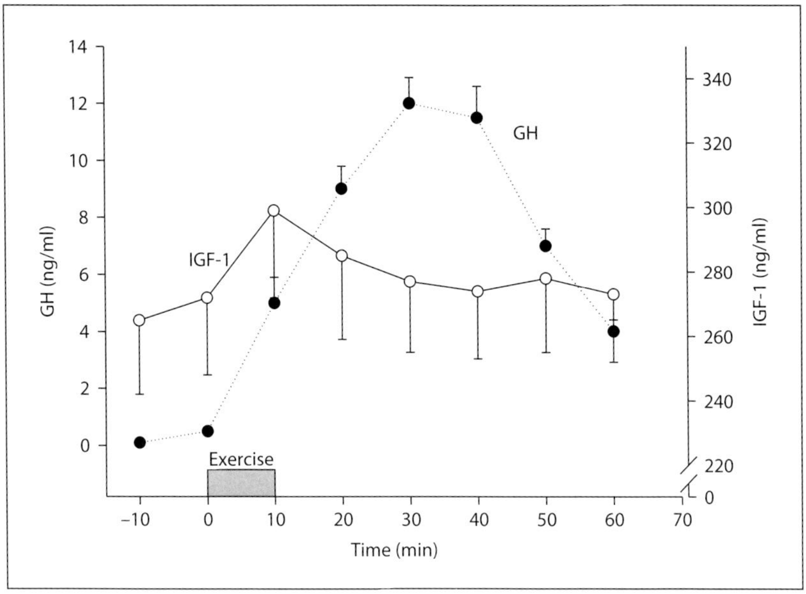

Fig. 1. Effect of aerobic exercise on GH and IGF-1 levels. The increase in IGF-1 occurs prior to the GH elevation suggesting that the exercise-induced increase in IGF-1 is GH-independent.

weight loss and/or improved fitness following exercise training programs in obese children and adolescents.

Insulin-Like Growth Factors

Several studies have demonstrated that acute exercise increases circulating IGF-1 levels. Interestingly, exercise-induced IGF-1 increase occurred following very short supra-maximal exercise (i.e. 90 s) [40], 10 min following the onset of endurance exercise [20, 41], and in exercise below and above the LAT [20]. Exercise also led to an increase in urinary IGF-1 [42].

The mechanism for this exercise-induced transient increase is not clearly understood. It is clear that the classic mechanism of increased hepatic IGF release due to exercise-induced secretion of GH is not the cause for IGF-1 release. GH increases mainly following high-intensity exercise, while IGF-1 increases after both low- and high-intensity exercise. In addition, circulating IGF-1 reaches its peak *before* the GH peak (i.e. 10 min compared to 30 min, fig. 1), while de novo hepatic IGF-1 synthesis and transport to the circulation, occurs several hours *after* administration of exogenous GH [43]. Moreover, exercise resulted in increases in IGF even in subjects with pituitary insufficiency [41]. These studies suggest that the exercise-associated increase in IGF-1 must reflect rapid changes in IGF-1 distribution in the circulation due to release from marginal pools or changes in IGF-1 removal, and is not GH-dependent.

The increase in circulating IGF-1 may result from its release from the exercising muscle. To test this, we performed a unilateral repeated wrist flexion against a relatively high resistance, and collected blood samples simultaneously during and post-exercise from the basilic vein of the exercising (representing local release) and resting arm (representing systemic response). We found a bilateral, simultaneous increase in IGF-1 suggesting that the local exercising muscle was not the source for of the IGF-1 increase [30].

Interestingly, Elias et al. [44] showed a transient rise in circulating IGF-1 immediately after an exercise test to exhaustion, followed by a significant drop to reach a nadir 60–90 min after the exercise, with gradual return to baseline levels. Consistent with this observation, prolonged and intense exercise sessions (1.5 h of intense soccer practice in children [45], or 1.5 h of wrestling practice in adolescents [46]) were associated with decreases in circulating IGF-1 levels. Interestingly, these sessions were also associated with increases in pro-inflammatory cytokines, and the authors suggested mediated the decrease in circulating IGF-1.

The effect of resistance exercise on circulating IGF-1 is inconsistent and has been studied mainly in adults. An increase in circulating IGF-1 and free IGF-1 following strength exercise was found by several investigators [47]. Moreover, eccentric exercise was associated with increases in muscle IGF-1 mRNA suggesting that IGF-1 may modulate tissue regeneration after mechanical damage [48]. Other studies found no change in circulating IGF-1 following heavy-resistance exercise [49], or even reduced IGF-1 levels the morning after high and moderate-intensity resistance workouts [50]. These conflicting results probably reflect differences in exercise protocols, timing of blood sampling, and individual fitness level, etc.

Insulin-Like Growth Factor-Binding Proteins

Several studies found increases in IGFBP-3 following endurance exercise [20, 51]. IGFBP-3 level measured by RIA increased with both low- and high-intensity exercise, and was greater during the above-LT protocol [20]. In contrast to the RIA measurements, IGFBP-3 measured by Western ligand blotting (WLB) did not change. A possible explanation for the discrepancy between RIA and WLB data was that the antibody used in the RIA recognizes both intact and fragment forms of IGFBP-3, while the WLB method measures only the intact IGFBP-3 form. Measurement of IGFBP-3 proteolysis rate as a function of exercise indicated that proteolysis occurred in the high-intensity exercise, and correlated with the peak increase in IGF-1 serum concentrations. It is important to note, however, that increases in IGFBP-3 proteolytic activity occurred in this study only for high-intensity exercise, while increases in IGFBP-3 and IGF-1 occurred for both low- and high-intensity exercise. Moreover, endurance exercise was not always associated with significant increase in IGF-1 proteolytic activity [52]. The mechanism for the increased IGFBP-3 proteolysis following high-intensity exercise may include changes in total and free ionized serum calcium [53], and/or serum and muscle acid-base changes [54].

Few studies have demonstrated changes in other IGFBPs following exercise including increases in IGFBP-1 [55, 56], and IGFBP-2 [49, 51]. The amount of these BPs in the circulation is much smaller compared to IGFBP-3, and they appear to play a smaller role in circulating IGF bioavailability. It is clear, however, that the exercise-induced effect on circulating IGF-1 is not only mediated by alteration of the amount of IGF-1 per se, but rather by the effect on its binding proteins.

Inflammatory Mediators

Several studies have demonstrated a significant increase of the pro-inflammatory cytokines IL-6, IL-1β and TNF-α following different types of exercise in adolescent males and females [46, 57]. Interestingly, the exercise in these studies was also associated with a significant increase in IL-1 receptor antagonist (IL-1ra), an anti-inflammatory mediator. A significant increase in IL-6, but not in IL-1ra, was also found following moderately-intense volleyball practice in elite male and female adolescent players. The finding of an increase only in IL-6 following relatively moderate-intensity volleyball training probably suggests that IL-6 is the most exercise-sensitive inflammatory cytokine.

The major source for the exercise-related IL-6 increase is believed to be the skeletal muscle [58]. IL-6 increases during exercise both with and without evidence of muscle damage. However, IL-6 is believed to play an important mediating role in the inflammatory response needed for exercise-associated muscle damage repair [59, 60]. It is possible that despite the moderate intensity, the frequent jumping and/or ball hitting and digging during a typical volleyball practice was associated with sub-clinical muscular and/or soft tissue damage that triggered a significant increase in circulating IL-6 levels.

One of the unique features of exercise is that it leads to a simultaneous increase of antagonistic mediators. As noted earlier, on the one hand, exercise stimulates anabolic components of the growth hormone (GH) → IGF-1 axis. On the other hand, exercise elevates catabolic pro-inflammatory cytokines such as IL-6, IL-1 and TNF-α. To make it even more complex, exercise may lead to a simultaneous increase of catabolic hormones like cortisol as well, and also to an increase in the anti-inflammatory cytokine IL-1ra. This indicates that several control mechanisms modulate the exercise response, and emphasizes the importance of optimal adaptation to the stimulation of exercise, particularly during adolescence. The very fine balance between the anabolic and inflammatory/catabolic response to exercise will determine the effectiveness of exercise training and the health consequences of exercise (fig. 2). If the anabolic response is

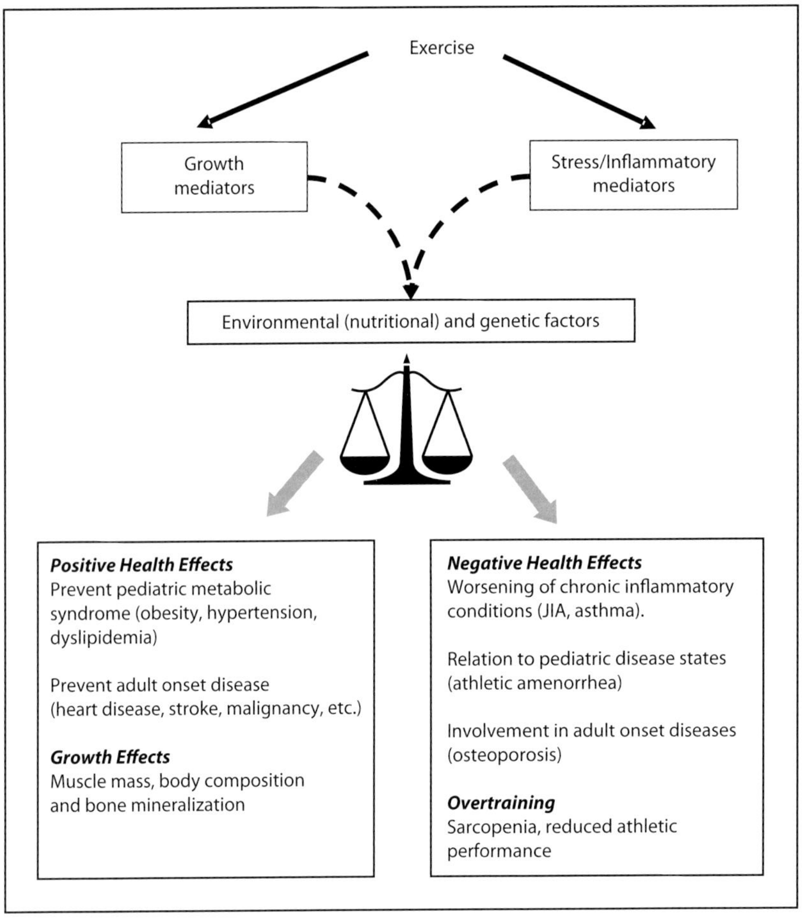

Fig. 2. Balance between exercise-associated increase in anabolic factors and inflammatory mediators.

stronger than the catabolic response, exercise will probably lead ultimately to increased muscle mass and improved fitness. A greater catabolic response, in particular if it persists for a long duration, may lead to overtraining. Therefore, changes in the anabolic-catabolic hormonal balance and in circulating inflammatory cytokines can be used by adolescent athletes and/or their coaches to gauge the training intensity in individual and team sports. The response of these mediators to different types of sports, training sessions or training protocols can be used as an objective tool to monitor the training load and to better plan training cycles throughout the competitive season (fig. 3).

It was believed that the source for the increase in circulating inflammatory cytokines was from the exercising muscle. To test this, we used the same trial of unilateral repeated wrist flexion against relatively high resistance, with simultaneous blood sample collection from the basilic vein of the exercising (representing local release)

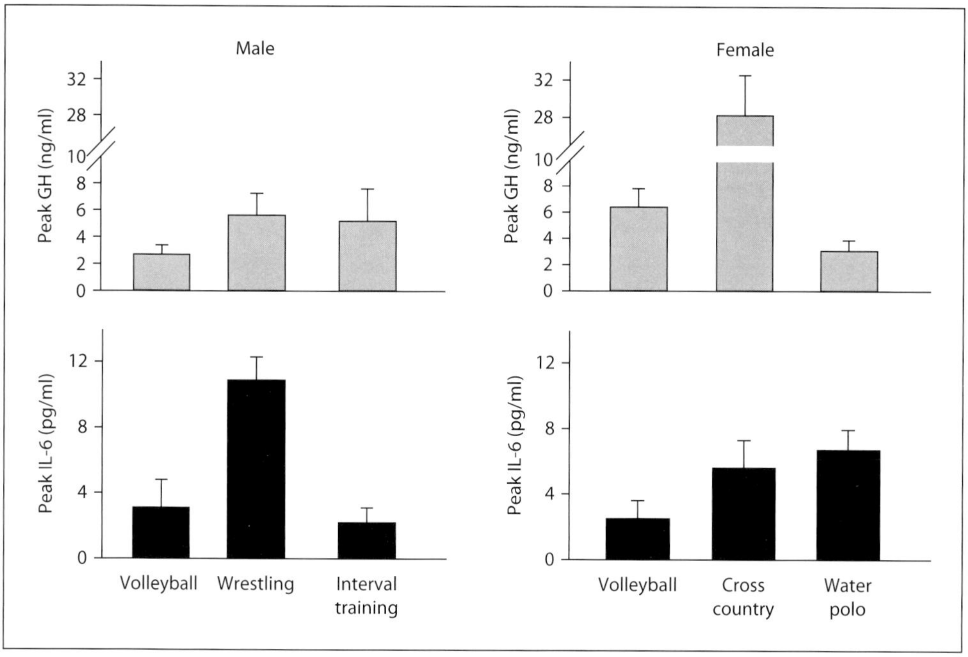

Fig. 3. Changes in IGF-1 (upper panel) and IL-6 levels (lower panel) following different types of exercise sessions in male (left panel) and female (right panel) adolescent athletes.

and resting arm (representing systemic response). Similar to the finding for IGF-1, there was a bilateral, simultaneous increase in the inflammatory cytokines suggesting that the local exercising muscle was not the source for of their increase [61]. The rapid exercise-induced increase in these cytokines must reflect circulatory distribution changes due to release from more available marginal pools.

Since it is believed that IL-6 plays a major role in hormonal response to exercise we tested the hypothesis that injection of rhIL-6 will lead to changes in the GH-IGF-1 that are similar to the responses induced by intense exercise in humans. Twelve healthy young adult volunteers were randomly assigned to receive rhIL-6 or saline for three hours. Plasma IL-6 levels during rhIL-6 infusion corresponded to the levels obtained during very strenuous exercise while no change in IL-6 levels were found in the controls. Recombinant human IL-6 induced significant increases in GH and a significant decrease in IGF-1 levels [62] (fig. 4). The results suggest that exogenous infusion of rhIL-6 without exercise induces a GH-IGF-1 axis response similar to that observed with strenuous exercise. The effect of intense exercise bouts (mediated at least partially by IL-6) is to initially create a metabolic state similar in some respects to a GH-resistant, catabolic state (increased GH with reduced IGF-1 level). Further studies are needed to clarify the exact role of inflammatory mediators in different types and less intense individual and team sports exercise.

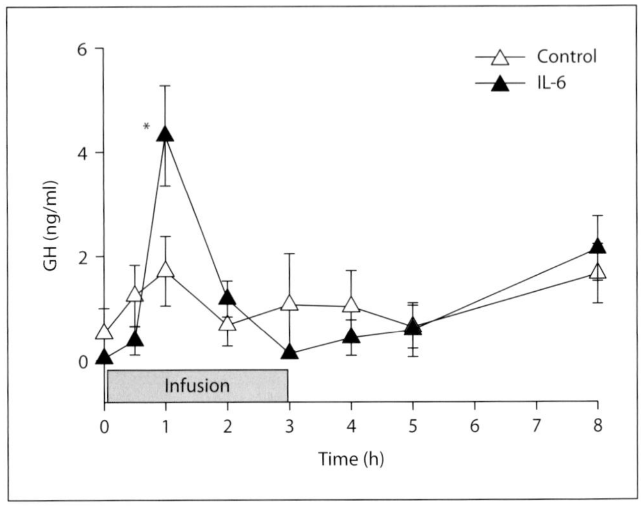

Fig. 4. Effect of rhIL-6 administration on GH secretion. Exogenous IL-6 administration mimics the physiological exercise-induced GH release.

Conclusions

The effectiveness of physical training depends on the training load and on the individual ability to tolerate it, and an imbalance between the two may lead to under- or overtraining. Therefore, many efforts have been made to find objective parameters to quantify the balance between training load and the athlete's tolerance, although with limited success. The complexity of hormonal responses to exercise has become increasingly apparent in recent years. Clearly, measurement of individual growth mediators can no longer suffice to gain an insight into mechanisms of growth regulation. This chapter suggests that the evaluation of exercise-induced changes in components of the GH-IGF-1 axis and inflammatory mediators, in particular in the growing adolescent athlete, may be used as an objective tool to assess the physical strain of training.

References

1 Krebs JM, Schneider VS, Evans H, Kuo MC, LeBlanc AD: Energy absorption, lean body mass, and total body fat changes during 5 weeks of continuous bed rest. Aviat Space Environ Med 1990;61:314–318.

2 Theintz GE, Howald H, Weiss U, Sizonenko PC: Evidence for a reduction of growth potential in adolescent female gymnasts. J Pediatr 1993;122:306–313.

3 Leung DW, Spencer SA, Cachianes G, Hammonds RG, Collins C, Henzel WJ, Barnard R, Waters MJ, Wood WI: Growth hormone receptor and serum binding protein: purification, cloning and expression. Nature 1987;330:537–543.

4 Berelowitz M, Szabo M, Frohman LA, Firestone S, Chu L, Hintz RL: Somatomedin-C mediates growth hormone negative feedback by effects on both the hypothalamus and the pituitary. Science 1981;212:1279–1281.

5 Rajaram S, Baylink DJ, Mohan S: Insulin-like growth factor-binding proteins in serum and other biological fluids: regulation and functions. Endocr Rev 1997;18:801–831.
6 Clark RG, Jansson JO, Isaksson O, Robinson IC: Intravenous growth hormone: growth responses to patterned infusions in hypophysectomized rats. J Endocrinol 1985;104:53–61.
7 Mauras N, Blizzard RM, Link K, Johnson ML, Rogol AD, Veldhuis JD: Augmentation of growth hormone secretion during puberty: evidence for a pulse amplitude-modulated phenomenon. J Clin Endocrinol Metab 1987;64:596–601.
8 Corpas E, Harman SM, Blackman MR: Human growth hormone and human aging. Endocr Rev 1993;14:20–39.
9 Merimee TJ, Zapf J, Froesch ER: Insulin-like growth factors in the fed and fasted states. J Clin Endocrinol Metab 1982;55:999–1002.
10 Ostrowski K, Rohde T, Asp S, Schjerling P, Pedersen BK: Pro- and anti-inflammatory cytokine balance in strenuous exercise in humans. J Physiol 1999;515:287–291.
11 Cooper DM, Radom-Aizik S, Schwindt C, Zaldivar F Jr: Dangerous exercise: lessons learned from dysregulated inflammatory responses to physical activity. J Appl Physiol 2007;103:700–709.
12 Eliakim A, Nemet D: Exercise provocation test for growth hormone secretion: methodologic considerations. Pediatr Exerc Sci 2008;20:370–378.
13 Buckler JM: Exercise as a screening test for growth hormone release. Acta Endocrinol (Copenh) 1972;69:219–229.
14 Felsing NE, Brasel JA, Cooper DM: Effect of low and high intensity exercise on circulating growth hormone in men. J Clin Endocrinol Metab 1992;75:157–162.
15 Sutton J, Lazarus L: Growth hormone in exercise: comparison of physiological and pharmacological stimuli. J Appl Physiol 1976;41:523–527.
16 Hartley LH, Mason JW, Hogan RP, Jones LG, Kotchen TA, Mougey EH, Wherry FE, Pennington LL, Ricketts PT: Multiple hormonal responses to graded exercise in relation to physical training. J Appl Physiol 1972;33:602–606.
17 Bar-Or O: Clinical implications of pediatric exercise physiology. Ann Clin Res 1982;14 Suppl 34:97–106.
18 Eliakim A, Brasel JA, Cooper DM: GH response to exercise: assessment of the pituitary refractory period, and relationship with circulating components of the GH-IGF-I axis in adolescent females. J Pediatr Endocrinol Metab 1999;12:47–55.
19 Wideman L, Weltman JY, Shah N, Story S, Veldhuis JD, Weltman A: Effects of gender on exercise-induced growth hormone release. J Appl Physiol 1999;87:1154–1162.
20 Schwarz AJ, Brasel JA, Hintz RL, Mohan S, Cooper DM: Acute effect of brief low- and high-intensity exercise on circulating insulin-like growth factor (IGF) I, II, and IGF-binding protein-3 and its proteolysis in young healthy men. J Clin Endocrinol Metab 1996;81:3492–3497.
21 Cappon J, Brasel JA, Mohan S, Cooper DM: Effect of brief exercise on circulating insulin-like growth factor I. J Appl Physiol 1994;76:2490–2496.
22 Kelijman M, Frohman LA: The role of the cholinergic pathway in growth hormone feedback. J Clin Endocrinol Metab 1991;72:1081–1087.
23 Casanueva FF, Villanueva L, Dieguez C, Diaz Y, Cabranes JA, Szoke B, Scanlon MF, Schally AV, Fernandez-Cruz A: Free fatty acids block growth hormone (GH) releasing hormone-stimulated GH secretion in man directly at the pituitary. J Clin Endocrinol Metab 1987;65:634–642.
24 Ronsen O, Haug E, Pedersen BK, Bahr R: Increased neuroendocrine response to a repeated bout of endurance exercise. Med Sci Sports Exerc 2001;33:568–575.
25 Kanaley JA, Weatherup-Dentes MM, Alvarado CR, Whitehead G: Substrate oxidation during acute exercise and with exercise training in lean and obese women. Eur J Appl Physiol 2001;85:68–73.
26 Stokes K, Nevill M, Frystyk J, Lakomy H, Hall G: Human growth hormone responses to repeated bouts of sprint exercise with different recovery periods between bouts. J Appl Physiol 2005;99:1254–1261.
27 Eliakim A, Portal S, Zadik Z, Rabinowitz J, dler-Portal D, Cooper DM, Zaldivar F, Nemet D: The effect of a volleyball practice on anabolic hormones and inflammatory markers in elite male and female adolescent players. J Strength Cond Res 2009;23:1553–1559.
28 Meckel Y, Eliakim A, Seraev M, Zaldivar F, Cooper DM, Sagiv M, Nemet D: The effect of a brief sprint interval exercise on growth factors and inflammatory mediators. J Strength Cond Res 2009;23:225–230.
29 Bailey RC, Olson J, Pepper SL, Porszasz J, Barstow TJ, Cooper DM: The level and tempo of children's physical activities: an observational study. Med Sci Sports Exerc 1995;27:1033–1041.
30 Eliakim A, Oh Y, Cooper DM: Effect of single wrist exercise on fibroblast growth factor-2, insulin-like growth factor, and growth hormone. Am J Physiol Regul Integr Comp Physiol 2000;279:R548–R553.
31 Cappon JP, Ipp E, Brasel JA, Cooper DM: Acute effects of high fat and high glucose meals on the growth hormone response to exercise. J Clin Endocrinol Metab 1993;76:1418–1422.

32 Waters DL, Qualls CR, Dorin R, Veldhuis JD, Baumgartner RN: Increased pulsatility, process irregularity, and nocturnal trough concentrations of growth hormone in amenorrheic compared to eumenorrheic athletes. J Clin Endocrinol Metab 2001;86: 1013–1019.
33 Eliakim A, Nemet D, Zaldivar F, McMurray RG, Culler FL, Galassetti P, Cooper DM: Reduced exercise-associated response of the GH-IGF-I axis and catecholamines in obese children and adolescents. J Appl Physiol 2006;100:1630–1637.
34 Blaak EE, Saris WHM: Substrate oxidation, obesity and exercise training. Best Pract Res Clin Endocrinol Metab 2002;16:667–678.
35 Brandou F, Dumortier M, Garandeau P, Mercier J, Brun JF: Effects of a two-month rehabilitation program on substrate utilization during exercise in obese adolescents. Diabetes Metab 2003;29:20–27.
36 Eliakim A, Beyth Y: Exercise training, menstrual irregularities and bone development in children and adolescents. J Pediatr Adolesc Gynecol 2003;16:201–206.
37 Lopes IM, Forga L, Martinez JA: Effects of leptin resistance on acute fuel metabolism after a high carbohydrate load in lean and overweight young men. J Am Coll Nutr 2001;20:643–648.
38 Patel L, Skinner AM, Price DA, Clayton PE: The influence of body mass index on growth hormone secretion in normal and short statured children. Growth Regul 1994;4:29–34.
39 Falk B, Sadres E, Constantini N, Zigel L, Lidor R, Eliakim A: The association between adiposity and the response to resistance training among pre- and early-pubertal boys. J Pediatr Endocrinol Metab 2002;15:597–606.
40 Kraemer WJ, Harman FS, Vos NH, Gordon SE, Nindl BC, Marx JO, Gomez AL, Volek JS, Ratamess NA, Mazzetti SA, Bush JA, Dohi K, Newton RU, Hakkinen K: Effects of exercise and alkalosis on serum insulin-like growth factor I and IGF-binding protein-3. Can J Appl Physiol 2000;25:127–138.
41 Bang P, Brandt J, Degerblad M, Enberg G, Kaijser L, Thoren M, Hall K: Exercise-induced changes in insulin-like growth factors and their low molecular weight binding protein in healthy subjects and patients with growth hormone deficiency. Eur J Clin Invest 1990;20:285–292.
42 De Palo EF, Gatti R, Lancerin F, De Palo CB, Cappellin E, Solda G, Spinella P: Effects of acute, heavy-resistance exercise on urinary peptide hormone excretion in humans. Clin Chem Lab Med 2003;41:1308–1313.
43 Marcus R, Butterfield G, Holloway L, Gilliland L, Baylink DJ, Hintz RL, Sherman BM: Effects of short term administration of recombinant human growth hormone to elderly people. J Clin Endocrinol Metab 1990;70:519–527.
44 Elias AN, Pandian MR, Wang L, Suarez E, James N, Wilson AF: Leptin and IGF-I levels in unconditioned male volunteers after short-term exercise. Psychoneuroendocrinology 2000;25:453–461.
45 Scheett TP, Mills PJ, Ziegler MG, Stoppani J, Cooper DM: Effect of exercise on cytokines and growth mediators in prepubertal children. Pediatr Res 1999; 46:429–434.
46 Nemet D, Oh Y, Kim HS, Hill M, Cooper DM: Effect of intense exercise on inflammatory cytokines and growth mediators in adolescent boys. Pediatrics 2002;110:681–689.
47 Bermon S, Ferrari P, Bernard P, Altare S, Dolisi C: Responses of total and free insulin-like growth factor-I and insulin-like growth factor binding protein-3 after resistance exercise and training in elderly subjects. Acta Physiol Scand 1999;165:51–56.
48 Bamman MM, Shipp JR, Jiang J, Gower BA, Hunter GR, Goodman A, McLafferty CL Jr, Urban RJ: Mechanical load increases muscle IGF-I and androgen receptor mRNA concentrations in humans. Am J Physiol Endocrinol Metab 2001;280:E383–E390.
49 Nindl BC, Kraemer WJ, Marx JO, Arciero PJ, Dohi K, Kellogg MD, Loomis GA: Overnight responses of the circulating IGF-I system after acute, heavy-resistance exercise. J Appl Physiol 2001;90:1319–1326.
50 Raastad T, Bjoro T, Hallen J: Hormonal responses to high- and moderate-intensity strength exercise. Eur J Appl Physiol 2000;82:121–128.
51 Chadan SG, Dill RP, Vanderhoek K, Parkhouse WS: Influence of physical activity on plasma insulin-like growth factor-1 and insulin-like growth factor binding proteins in healthy older women. Mech Age Dev 1999;109:21–34.
52 Dall R, Lange KH, Kjaer M, Jorgensen JO, Christiansen JS, Orskov H, Flyvbjerg A: No evidence of insulin-like growth factor-binding protein 3 proteolysis during a maximal exercise test in elite athletes. J Clin Endocrinol Metab 2001;86:669–674.
53 Lamson G, Giudice LC, Cohen P, Liu F, Gargosky S, Muller HL, Oh Y, Wilson KF, Hintz RL, Rosenfeld RG: Proteolysis of IGFBP-3 may be a common regulatory mechanism of IGF action in vivo. Growth Regul 1993;3:91–95.
54 Martin JL, Baxter RC: Insulin-like growth factor-binding protein from human plasma: purification and characterization. J Biol Chem 1986;261:8754–8760.

55 Suikkari AM, Sane T, Seppala M, Yki-Jarvinen H, Karonen SL, Koivisto VA: Prolonged exercise increases serum insulin-like growth factor-binding protein concentrations. J Clin Endocrinol Metab 1989;68:141–144.
56 Hopkins NJ, Jakeman PM, Hughes SC, Holly JM: Changes in circulating insulin-like growth factor-binding protein-1 (IGFBP-1) during prolonged exercise: effect of carbohydrate feeding. J Clin Endocrinol Metab 1994;79:1887–1890.
57 Nemet D, Rose-Gottron CM, Mills PJ, Cooper DM: Effect of water polo practice on cytokines, growth mediators, and leukocytes in girls. Med Sci Sports Exerc 2003;35:356–363.
58 Keller P, Keller C, Carey AL, Jauffred S, Fischer CP, Steensberg A, Pedersen BK: Interleukin-6 production by contracting human skeletal muscle: autocrine regulation by IL-6. Biochem Biophys Res Commun 2003;310:550–554.
59 Steensberg A, Keller C, Starkie RL, Osada T, Febbraio MA, Pedersen BK: IL-6 and TNF-alpha expression in, and release from, contracting human skeletal muscle. Am J Physiol Endocrinol Metab 2002;283:E1272–E1278.
60 Pedersen BK, Steensberg A, Fischer C, Keller C, Ostrowski K, Schjerling P: Exercise and cytokines with particular focus on muscle-derived IL-6. Exerc Immunol Rev 2001;7:18–31.
61 Nemet D, Hong S, Mills PJ, Ziegler MG, Hill M, Cooper DM: Systemic vs. local cytokine and leukocyte responses to unilateral wrist flexion exercise. J Appl Physiol 2002;93:546–554.
62 Nemet D, Eliakim A, Zaldivar F, Cooper DM: Effect of rhIL-6 infusion on GH->IGF-I axis mediators in humans. Am J Physiol Regul Integr Comp Physiol 2006;291:R1663–R1668.

Dan Nemet, MD
Child Health and Sports Center
Pediatric Department, Meir General Hospital
Kfar-Saba, Israel 44821
Tel. +972 9 7472134, Fax +972 9 7471303, E-Mail dnemet@gmail.com

Jürimäe J, Hills AP, Jürimäe T (eds): Cytokines, Growth Mediators and Physical Activity in Children during Puberty.
Med Sport Sci. Basel, Karger, 2010, vol 55, pp 156–173

Effect of Acute and Chronic Exercise on Ghrelin and Adipocytokines during Pubertal Development

Robert R. Kraemer[a] · V. Daniel Castracane[b]

[a]Department of Kinesiology and Health Studies, Southeastern Louisiana University, Hammond, La., and
[b]Department of Obstetrics and Gynecology, Texas Tech University School of Medicine at the Permian Basin, Odessa, Tex., USA

Abstract

It is important to understand the factors that regulate the development of obesity during adolescence due to the increased risk of adult obesity, metabolic syndrome and the deleterious health effects of early puberty which may increase the risk of breast cancer later in life. Leptin, ghrelin, and adiponectin are peptides that affect energy homeostasis and insulin action. Similar to findings in adults, steady-state exercise does not change leptin concentrations and aerobic training without a change in body weight. A small amount of available data suggest that acute exercise does not increase circulating adiponectin concentrations in adolescents; however, it is very possible that more rigorous exercise protocols could acutely affect circulating adiponectin levels. Training studies indicate that shorter lengths of exercise training have a stronger effect on increases in adiponectin concentrations in male than female adolescents. It appears that if training is extended, increases in adiponectin levels will accompany improvements in insulin sensitivity. There are no studies of acute or chronic exercise on high-molecular weight adiponectin in adolescents and since this is thought to be the bioactive form of adiponectin, these studies are definitely needed. Investigations have demonstrated that exercise training increases total ghrelin levels in adolescents and that ghrelin is sensitive to reductions in body fat or increases in energy expenditure in this population. These findings are similar to those in adults. Moreover, there is evidence that luteinizing hormone is a predictor of total ghrelin levels in girls and suggests that ghrelin is a biomarker of energy imbalance across the menstrual cycle.

In 1994, the prototypical adipokine, leptin, was discovered after isolation of the *ob* gene [1]. As a satiety hormone its presence led to considerable interest and many studies [2]. Since that time, a number of appetite hormones, both adipokines and enterokines, have been discovered, and their effects and signaling potential investigated. These include but are not limited to, ghrelin, obestatin, orexin, peptide YY (PYY), and adiponectin. During this period of appetite hormone discovery, the prevalence of obesity and metabolic syndrome has risen substantially in industrialized countries around the world, with increased childhood obesity rates of particular concern [3]. A number of studies have provided epidemiological as well as experimental human and animal model data that indicate overnutrition in early life leads to obesity, glucose intolerance, hypertension, and dyslipidemia [4]. Additionally, there is evidence that early life events may have long-term adverse effects on adipose tissue and its synthesis of hormones, enzymes and growth factors, ultimately resulting in molecular and cellular changes that lead to increased adiposity [5]. Moreover, substantial evidence points toward the importance of physical activity in providing protection from adolescent obesity [6–8]. As such, the need for understanding the role that these hormones play in maintaining health in adolescents has become increasingly important.

A number of studies have examined the effects of exercise on alterations in appetite hormones [2, 9]. Although some data exist on a number of appetite peptides, most of the work in this area has been conducted on leptin, ghrelin, and adiponectin; thus these peptides will be the focus of this chapter. Many studies have involved laboratory animals as well as adult patients with obesity and anorexia nervosa. Much fewer data exist regarding younger populations. This presents a significant research void at a time when development of childhood obesity is increasing as is the need for interventions to address this major health issue. Without understanding how appetite and exercise are integrally affected, interventions cannot be developed to substantially correct this situation and prevent life-long health problems for many individuals.

In this chapter, we present background information on leptin, ghrelin, and adiponectin. This is followed by a description of exercise studies involving the effects of acute exercise on the appetite hormone with comparison of findings in adults to that of adolescents. A subsequent discussion of studies regarding the effects of chronic exercise on the appetite hormones will compare findings in adults to those in adolescents.

Leptin

In 1950, with the discovery of the mutant obese mouse model (ob/ob), investigations into the regulation of obesity in this mutation were initiated. When the obese mouse was parabiosed (a linking of bodies and a sharing of the two vascular supplies) to the normal-weight (NW) mouse, the former became lean, indicating that some substance from the lean mouse crossed through the shared vascular connection to result in this weight loss. It was also apparent that the obese mouse was deficient in some (hormonal) substance [10]. It subsequently took more than 40 years until the discovery of the missing substance, leptin, the 16-kDa satiety peptide produced in adipocytes. This finding led to the important observation that adipose tissue serves as an endocrine gland and that leptin levels are proportional to the amount of body fat [8]. Further work determined that the effect of circulating leptin on satiety was through its hypothalamic regulation of the orexigenic neurotransmitter, neuropeptide Y (NPY) and stimulation of hypothalamic anorectic peptide, α-melanocortin-stimulating hormone [11]. The important early observation that leptin administration could result in weight loss in the obese mouse, led to great interest in leptin as the hormone which might 'cure' obesity. Several studies revealed that leptin was not effective in reducing body weight when administered to individuals with obesity and the suggestion that there might be a state of 'leptin resistance' became entrenched in the obesity literature.

With greater fat mass, leptin expression and thus circulating leptin levels are higher than in leaner humans [12]. Moreover, the expression of leptin in humans is sexually dimorphic with greater leptin levels in females than in males [12]. It has been proposed that gender differences in the expression of leptin may be due to the inhibition of leptin by androgens, stimulation of leptin by estrogens, and gender differences in adipocyte deposition [13, 14]. Interestingly, increased circulating leptin levels occur at a time that coincides with the onset of menarche in girls [15]. These differences are maintained in older, normally cycling women [12] and leptin levels decline in hypogonadal men after administration of testosterone [16, 17]. There is cross-sectional data from the authors' group, however, to suggest that gender and estrogen treatment differences in relation to serum leptin are due to differences in body composition and not circulating estrogen [18].

Long and short forms of the leptin receptor are expressed in the arcuate, ventromedial, and dorsomedial hypothalamic nuclei [19], allowing these tissues to respond to leptin and regulate energy balance (EB) [13]. Central administration of leptin appears to stimulate lipolysis in adipose tissue and hepatic fatty acid uptake and oxidation [20], confirming the importance of the central action of leptin. Additionally, there is now evidence that under conditions of elevated circulating lipids, leptin resistance occurs. Specifically, there are data demonstrating that overnutrition increases inflammatory cytokines and elevates free fatty acid levels which induce endoplasmic reticulum stress in leptin receptors expressing hypothalamic neurons, reducing leptin sensitivity in the mouse [21]. Comparable studies in humans remain to be conducted. Reduction in factors that enhance endoplasmic reticulum stress results in improvement in leptin sensitivity in these hypothalamic neurons. As such, exercise is a counter factor for overnutrition, elevated inflammatory cytokines at rest, and plasma free fatty acid levels, and may have a positive effect on leptin resistance.

The importance in understanding factors regulating development of obesity during adolescence lies in the higher risk of adult obesity and metabolic syndrome [22]. Moreover, adolescent obesity is accompanied by increased circulating leptin levels that activate the HPA-axis and produce the additional deleterious health effect of early puberty which may increase the risk of breast cancer later in life [22, 23]. Thus, intervention prior to puberty with newly developed strategies that affect the mechanisms of adolescent obesity warrant increased attention.

An additional health concern in adolescence is amenorrhea. The most common cause of amenorrhea in adolescents originates in the hypothalamus, indicating an alteration in the hypothalamic-pituitary-gonadal axis [24]. Leptin provides EB information via leptin receptors in the hypothalamus (close to the median eminence) to regulate food intake. There is evidence that leptin influences hypothalamic gonadotropin-releasing hormone (GnRH) secretion which ultimately stimulates the luteinizing hormone (LH) surge, follicle-stimulating hormone (FSH) release and stimulation of the ovarian follicle, and subsequent estrogen production [24]. Hypoleptinemia, resulting from inadequate energy intake or decreased adipose tissue mass, may compensate for elevated energy expenditure in active female adolescent athletes [25] and result in adolescent amenorrhea, having potential deleterious effects on development of bone mass. Interestingly, in a study of women with hypothalamic amenorrhea who were actively exercising or had lost considerable weight, a three-month regimen of recombinant leptin improved function of the hypothalamic-pituitary-gonadal (HPG) axis [26]. In summary, this information points to the importance of understanding the role of leptin in order to treat and maintain adolescent health.

Exercise and Leptin in Adults

Adult Exercise Response Studies in Adults

A number of studies have examined the effect of acute exercise on leptin levels in adult populations. Factors that may have an effect on leptin concentrations following exercise include: (1) the circadian rhythm of leptin; (2) energy expended during the exercise bout; (3) resting leptin levels; (4) gender, and (5) postprandial time prior to exercise. We have reported that leptin levels are reduced in response to exercise in older women after an overnight fast [27], but that these reductions were due to normal circadian rhythm reductions in leptin and not exercise per se. In other investigations, we have demonstrated no effect of hormone replacement therapy on leptin responses to exercise in older women [27], nor any effect of different exercise intensities on acute leptin responses in young men [28]. Weltman et al. [29] also reported no change in leptin levels in response to 30 min of exercise in young men, regardless of different exercise intensities, and these subjects were 13 h postprandial. Others have also demonstrated declines in men in response to exercise [30]; however, Fisher et al. [31] showed increases in circulating leptin in men when a standard meal preceded a 41-minute bout of exercise. With regard to energy expenditure, it has been shown that negative EB induced by exercise and inadequate caloric intake, not exercise per se, leads to disruption of leptin pulsatility [25]. Suppression of GnRH, which disrupts the HPG axis, is mediated by a deficiency of leptin [24]. With respect to males, energy imbalance has also been shown to alter leptin in young men with exercise-induced negative EB reducing 24-hour leptin levels and positive EB causing an increase [32]. Together, these studies demonstrate the importance of leptin as a signal of energy status in maintaining the health of the individual.

Exercise Training Studies in Adults

A number of training studies have been conducted to determine the effects of chronic exercise on circulating leptin. We examined the effect of 9 weeks of aerobic exercise training on leptin levels in middle-aged women with obesity. Women trained 3–4 days per week and after 9 weeks, cardiorespiratory fitness levels, body weight and body fat had not changed significantly, nor were leptin levels altered [33]. In a study of young males with type 2 diabetes, 1 month of cycling exercise and diet modification led to reduced body weight and leptin levels [34]. In a 2-month training (walking, jogging, stair climbing) study of postmenopausal women on and off hormone replacement therapy, fat loss was associated with reductions in leptin concentrations regardless of whether subjects received hormone replacement therapy [35]. Another investigation determined resting levels and acute leptin responses to graded exercise before and after a 20-week cycle training program in men and women. Adjusting for loss of fat mass accounted for training-induced changes in resting levels; there were no training-induced alterations in leptin response to exercise [36]. Collectively, these studies suggest that training which results in reductions in fat mass will reduce circulating leptin.

Leptin and Exercise in Adolescents

With regard to leptin response to acute exercise in adolescents, we examined the effect of acute intense exercise on changes in leptin levels in adolescent female athletes over the course of a short cross-country season [37]. All subjects had a history of menstrual cycles although, as is typical for this age, they were a somewhat erratic. All were tested in a 4.5-hour postprandial state and completed graded exercise tests to exhaustion at baseline, 4 weeks, and completion of the 7-week training season. Leptin levels increased in response to the different graded exercise tests (fig. 1). Interestingly, cortisol levels also increased, which have been shown to promote leptin production [2]. In a study of male adolescents, Pomerants et al. [38] investigated ghrelin and leptin responses to acute cycling in 60 boys at different stages of puberty. Prepubertal children had greater serum ghrelin levels than older children, i.e. Tanner stages II and III. Ghrelin and leptin levels did not change significantly with 30 min of cycling at ~95% of ventilatory threshold although insulin declined. This occurred, regardless of the fact that subjects consumed a light, standard lunch 2–3 h prior to exercise. The discrepancies in these findings and the increases found in the previously mentioned study [37] may be due to the lower exercise intensity used. Results of the study indicated that there are no changes in ghrelin and leptin in response to moderately intense aerobic exercise in young boys regardless of the pubertal stages of development. Souza et al. [39] examined the effect of a maximal aerobic exercise test on untrained children and adolescents (6–11 years of age) with obesity. Leptin levels did not increase in response to the

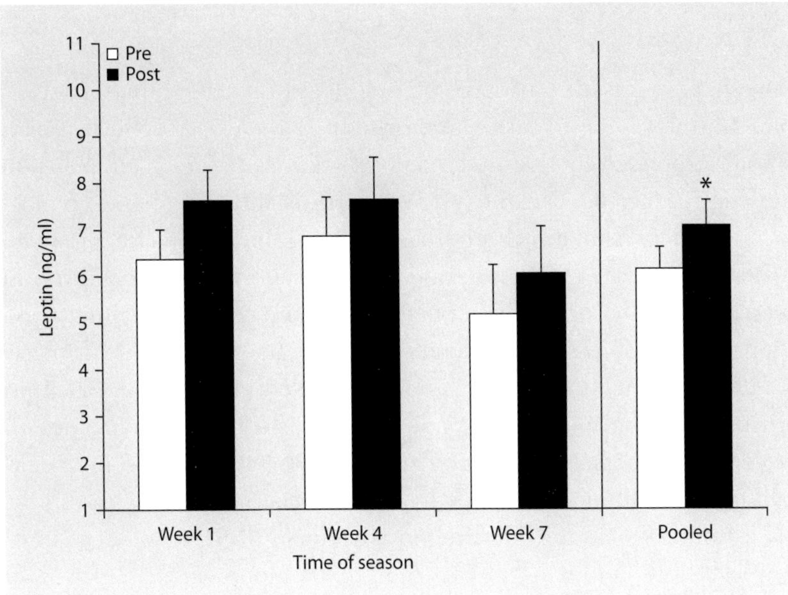

Fig. 1. Data represent mean (± SEM) leptin concentrations before (Pre) and after (Post) graded exercise test for weeks 1, 4 and 7 of the training season as well as pooled means. * Significantly different than Pre value. Reprinted from Kraemer et al. [37], with permission.

graded exercise test. Elloimi et al. [40] conducted a 2-month weight loss intervention on adolescent boys with obesity (BMI = 30.8). Subjects completed one of three conditions: (1) energy restriction; (2) exercise training that corresponded with the point at which there was maximal lipid oxidation, or (3) energy restriction and training.

The adolescents in the energy restriction and exercise training group lost body fat, increased plasma adiponectin by 74%, reduced plasma leptin levels by 38% and had a lower HOMA value (measure of insulin sensitivity). Moreover, their adiponectin/leptin ratio was higher than in the other two groups. Conclusions were that training with energy restriction normalizes leptin and adiponectin levels and improves insulin sensitivity. Kelly et al. [41] investigated the effects of eight weeks of aerobic training on adipokines in overweight children (Tanner stage II). There was no weight loss in the subjects and no concomitant change in circulating leptin levels. These findings are similar to those in the adult population and suggest that weight loss is important in modifying the leptin profile.

In summary, acute exercise has been shown to increase or not change circulating leptin concentrations in adolescents in response to graded exercise. Discrepant results need to be elucidated with future studies. Steady-state exercise has been shown to not change leptin concentrations similar to findings in adults. Aerobic training that induces reductions in body weight/fat is associated with reductions in circulating leptin levels.

Adiponectin

Another adipokine that has raised considerable interest and is found in high concentrations in human plasma (5–30 μg/ml) is adiponectin [42]. Adiponectin is a 244-amino acid hormone expressed by the *apM1* gene in adipose tissue. It circulates in several forms; the high-molecular weight (HMW) form is thought to be the most effective in endocrinological regulation and tissue signaling and involves at least two receptors, AdipoR1 and AdipoR2 [43]. Adiponectin reduces free fatty acid levels in the blood that would normally increase after eating [44] and reduces hepatic blood glucose production [45, 46]. Diet-induced hyperinsulinemia and dyslipidemia have been shown to reduce adiponectin content in skeletal muscle [47] which is thought to be related to insulin resistance. Moreover, adiponectin concentrations increase in response to thiazoledinedione treatment, which may indicate it is an important mechanism for thiazolidinedione-induced increase in insulin sensitivity [48]. Conversely, pro-inflammatory cytokines such as tumor necrosis factor-α (TNF-α) reduce circulating adiponectin levels [46] and it is known that TNF-α, along with circulation of excessive lipids, contribute to the development of metabolic syndrome as well as cardiovascular disease [49]. Moreover, adolescents with type 2 diabetes have been shown to have reduced insulin sensitivity along with increased soleus IL-6 and reduced circulating adiponectin [50].

Acute rigorous exercise is known to elicit concentration increases in the inflammation responsive cytokines, IL-6 [50] and TNF-α in adults [51]and similarly, there is evidence that rigorous exercise (a 1.5-hour soccer practice) produces a sharp increase in IL-6 and TNF-α in 8- to 11-year-old children [52]. With rigorous exercise training, however, there is a downregulation of blood monocyte TNF-α-stimulated cytokine release [53]. Moreover, acute exercise is known to increase insulin sensitivity, major mechanisms being increased oxidation of fatty acid and inhibition of hepatic glucose production [54]. Collectively, these effects of acute and chronic exercise on metabolism closely related to factors associated with adiponectin, indicate that adiponectin is altered with some forms of exercise in adults and in children, and could play an important role in improving insulin sensitivity.

Acute Exercise and Adiponectin in Adults

In adults, adiponectin responses to exercise have been investigated using different exercise modes, intensities and durations. The present authors determined the exercise responses to adiponectin under two conditions [55]. In the first condition, male subjects exercised for 30 min on a treadmill at ~80% of VO_{2max}. In the second condition, male runners completed a similar duration of exercise, but at 60, 75, 90 and 100% of VO_{2max}. Compared with a control trial, circulating glucose concentrations did not change in the first experiment but did in the second experiment. Both conditions elicited increases in circulating adiponectin, but these increases could be accounted for by hemoconcentration or normal postprandial diurnal changes. These findings in adults have been confirmed by other investigators in response to 60 min of cycling at 65% VO_{2max} [56] and 2 h of exercise at 50% VO_{2max} in fasting and nonfasting conditions [57]. Higher intensities for prolonged periods have been shown to acutely reduce adiponectin. Jürimäe et al. [58] reported that completion of a 6,000-meter rowing ergometer test by well-trained athletes elicited a significant reduction in adiponectin levels even after correcting for plasma volume shifts. Recently, however, it was reported that an hour of cycling at 50% of VO_{2max} did not affect the levels of HMW adiponectin, nor the HMW to total adiponectin ratio in healthy men [59]. There are data indicating that obese adolescents with fatty liver disease respond to a glucose tolerance test with declining HMW and total adiponectin levels [60].

Acute Exercise and Adiponectin in Adolescents

Very little data exist regarding the effects of acute exercise on circulating adiponectin levels in adolescents. A recent study investigated the effects of two acute 75-min bouts of exercise on catecholamine and adiponectin concentrations in children, aged 8–17 years, with type 1 diabetes on an insulin pump. Adiponectin levels did not change significantly during exercise nor were adiponectin concentrations related to changes in epinephrine concentrations, however, children/adolescents with higher adiponectin levels were more likely to develop exercise-induced hypoglycemia [61].

Exercise Training Effects in Adolescents

A number of investigators have examined the effects of exercise training on adolescents. A study of nonobese American middle-school aged children before and at the end of the school year that included a school-based fitness program, revealed improvements in VO_{2max}, body composition, homeostasis mode assessment (HOMA-IR), and increases in adiponectin concentrations [62]. In another training study, Elloumi et al. [63] found that adolescent boys with obesity completing a two-month individualized exercise training program coupled with energy restriction showed improvements in body composition along with increases in plasma adiponectin and reductions in leptin. The training program also led to improvement in the rate of lipid oxidation and lower HOMA-IR scores indicating better insulin sensitivity. An investigation of the effects of six weeks of training on Korean adolescent males using jump-rope as an exercise modality, reported improvement in insulin sensitivity and circulating adiponectin concentrations without concomitant changes in inflammatory cytokines IL-6 and TNF-α [64].

Studies on female adolescents with obesity suggest, however, that more training is required to elicit similar adiponectin adaptations found in male adolescents with obesity. Forty-four adolescent girls with obesity completed either a 12-week program which included lifestyle modification and exercise, or served as a control group. The lifestyle modification and exercise group demonstrated reductions in body weight and body fat that was accompanied by reduced resting systolic blood pressure, HOMA-IR and leptin. However, adiponectin concentrations did not change significantly [65]. Another 12-week training study also reported improvements in insulin sensitivity but no changes in circulating adiponectin or IL-6 in adolescent girls with overweight or obesity conditions [66]. In a study of 27 adolescent patients with obesity, who completed 2 months of diet and exercise, the young women improved in ability to oxidize lipids and this improvement was positively correlated with post-training adiponectin levels [67]. In a longer study of obese Japanese adolescent girls, subjects completed aerobic training exercises 4–5 days per week for 7 months. These girls lost body weight and percentage fat which was accompanied by improvements in VO_{2max} and adiponectin levels and reductions in circulating leptin [68]. Weight loss seems essential to the decrease in adiponectin.

The little evidence that exists suggests that acute exercise does not increase circulating adiponectin concentrations in adolescents; however, it is possible that more rigorous exercise protocols could acutely affect circulating adiponectin levels. Training studies suggest that shorter lengths of exercise training have a stronger effect on increases in adiponectin in male adolescents than female adolescents. It appears that if training is extended, there will be increases in adiponectin levels that will accompany improvements in insulin sensitivity. There are no studies of acute or chronic exercise on HMW adiponectin in adolescents and since this is thought to be the bioactive form of adiponectin, these studies are definitely needed.

Ghrelin

The endogenous ligand for the growth hormone secretogogue receptor (GHS-R) stomach was purified in 1999 from the stomach and named ghrelin [69]. It is found in the acylated as well as nonacylated (desacyl ghrelin) forms in the blood with greater concentrations of the latter [69]. The acylated form is known to bind to the GHS-R1-a receptor whereas the desacyl ghrelin form does not. However, recent evidence demonstrates that acylated as well as desacyl ghrelin stimulates the C2CI2 skeletal muscle myoblast indicating the possibility of an unknown receptor for the nonacylated form [70]. Released in greater concentrations during fasting, ghrelin transmits a peripheral hunger signal to the central nervous system [71]. Although it is mainly produced and released from the stomach, with more ghrelin-producing cells in the fundus than pylorus, it is also found in the duodenum, jejunum, ileum, and colon, with declining concentrations in these tissues [72–75]. Moreover, ghrelin's presence

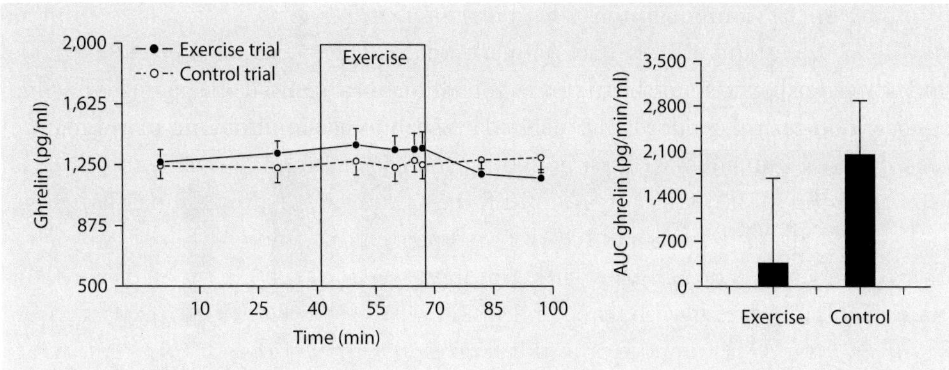

Fig. 2. Left: Data depict mean ± SE ghrelin concentrations for exercise and control trials before exercise, after each exercise intensity, and for 30 min of recovery. Concentrations are for 40 and 10 min before exercise; after each exercise intensity (10 min of 60% VO_{2max}, 10 min of 75% VO_{2max}, 5 min at 90% VO_{2max}, and 2 min at 100% VO_{2max}), and 15 and 30 min of recovery. Right. Values are area under the curve (AUC) concentrations for ghrelin. Reprinted from Kraemer et al. [88], with permission.

has been identified in other tissues including the pancreas, testis, placenta, lung, cardiomyocytes, chondrocytes, and lymphocytes [76–79].

Ghrelin's orexigenic effect is produced through stimulation of hypothalamic arcuate nucleus neurons in the hypothalamus [80], causing increases in expression of NPY and agouti-related peptide (AgRP) [81, 82]. Interestingly, the orexigenic effect of ghrelin is absent in NPY and AgRP knockout mice [83]. As such, feeding regulates the daily pattern of ghrelin with circulating concentrations increasing before meals and declining after feeding [84, 85]. Both the presence of food in the stomach and the postprandial rise in insulin have been implicated in the postprandial decline in ghrelin. Administration of ghrelin increases GH release in rats and humans with a potency to stimulate GH release three times greater than growth hormone-releasing hormone [86, 87].

Ghrelin and Exercise in Adults

Adult Acute Response Studies

The present authors have investigated the effects of acute exercise on total ghrelin concentrations and have reported no changes in response to rigorous treadmill running in young males, although GH concentrations rose sharply [88] (fig. 2). In this study, however, the present authors determined that ghrelin was associated with insulin-growth factor-1 (IGF-1), the growth factor stimulated by GH release, as well as IGFBP-3, an important binding protein for IGF-1 that affects its biological activity,

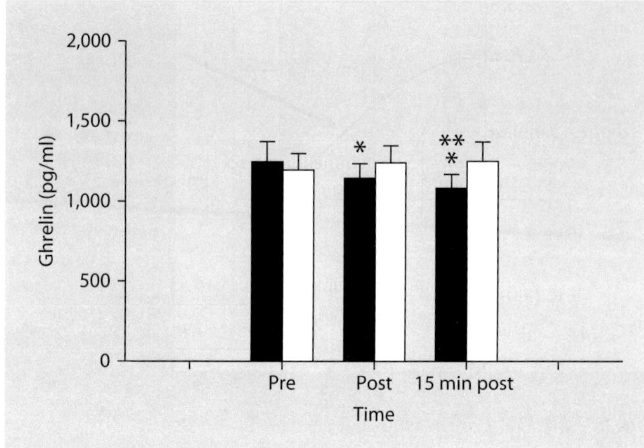

Fig. 3. Ghrelin responses for concentric (solid) and eccentric (hatched) trials before exercise, immediately after exercise, and after 15 min of recovery. Values are mean ± SE. * $p < 0.05$ compared with pre-exercise value for concentric trials; ** $p < 0.05$ compared with postexercise value for concentric trial. Reprinted from Kraemer et al. [91], with permission.

but not growth hormone. Another study investigated GH and ghrelin responses to low, moderate, and high intensity treadmill bouts [89] and also reported no changes in total ghrelin concentrations. In an investigation that manipulated feeding status, subjects performed 15 min of cycling at a low-to-moderate workload of 150 W. They reported no changes in total ghrelin levels in response to exercise regardless of whether it was in a fed or fasted state [90]. In another study from the present authors' group, the effects of resistance exercise on changes in GH and ghrelin were investigated [91] (fig. 3). Here, the present authors isolated the forms of muscle action so that in one trial, young men performed concentric (muscle shortening) contractions only whereas during a separate trial, eccentric (muscle lengthening) contractions only were performed. Interestingly, the concentric but not the eccentric muscle contractions were associated with lower circulating ghrelin concentrations. There are sparse data regarding the effects of exercise on both acylated and desacylated ghrelin. Broom et al. [92] investigated the effects of 1 h of running at 72% VO_{2max} on acylated ghrelin concentrations. They found that total ghrelin levels did not change with exercise however, acylated ghrelin was suppressed, suggesting that future studies should determine both acylated and desacylated forms of ghrelin. The same research group subsequently compared the effects of both resistance (90 min) and aerobic exercise (1 h) using a research design that included standardized meals and hunger ratings during and after the exercise [93].

Findings concerning exercise-induced reduction in acylated ghrelin and appetite suggested that reductions in appetite following exercise were due to suppressed acylated ghrelin. Since acylated ghrelin comprises a smaller portion of the total ghrelin concentration, these results suggest that studies revealing reduced total ghrelin in response to exercise may be due to large changes in acylated ghrelin. Collectively, these studies suggest that acute aerobic exercise results in no changes in ghrelin unless exercise volume is such that large caloric expenditure occurs and that resistance exercise will suppress total ghrelin concentrations. Moreover, acylated ghrelin appears to be more affected by exercise than total ghrelin.

Adult Exercise Training Studies

Training studies in patients with obesity suggest that weight loss is associated with increases in total ghrelin concentrations. A caloric restriction and exercise study of overweight men and women revealed increases in total ghrelin after caloric restriction and following caloric restriction plus exercise [94]. A study of 173 overweight postmenopausal women who completed a year of aerobic training and lost weight which was associated with increased total ghrelin levels [95]. Other investigators have reported much higher total ghrelin levels in amenorrheic women compared with sedentary as well as ovulating and exercising women. Conversely, in a study of men and women with obesity in which short weight-loss/exercise programs were used to investigate effects on appetite hormones, no change in total ghrelin levels were reported [96]. Other researchers who have used longer training programs with a greater effect on body composition have reported increases in total ghrelin levels in subjects with obesity who have lost weight. Thus, long-term exercise training typically increases total ghrelin levels in adults.

Ghrelin and Exercise in Children

Adolescents Acute Response Studies

Investigations of the effect of acute exercise on ghrelin responses in children have typically reported no alterations in total ghrelin levels. Pomerants et al. [97] conducted a study with 60 young male subjects at different stages of puberty who completed 30 min of cycling at an exercise intensity just below their previously determined ventilatory threshold. Although baseline total ghrelin levels were higher for the pre-pubertal participants as compared with the Tanner stage II and III subjects, total ghrelin levels were not changed by cycling exercise in any of the groups. In a study of 17 overweight and 17 NW male adolescent boys, aerobic exercise (walking, jogging, cycling, stair climbing) at 65–75% of maximal heart rate reserve was performed for 1 h each day for 5 consecutive days and acylated as well as total ghrelin was measured [98]. The investigators reported lower fasting total ghrelin levels in overweight boys compared to NW boys and that exercise did not affect total ghrelin concentrations in either group. However, acylated ghrelin concentrations were elevated following exercise and this increase was greater in the NW than the overweight boys. Moreover, greater acylated ghrelin concentrations were associated with greater appetite in the young males.

These results emphasize the point that that acylated ghrelin may represent the more important form and is too often ignored in many studies.

Adolescent Exercise Training Studies

With regard to training studies, Nitsche et al. [99] investigated the effects of a very short (10 days) exercise training program with a hypocaloric diet in overweight (BMI = 26.8) children (13.1 years). The intervention produced a reduction in BMI and a tendency for ghrelin and the respiratory quotient to increase, which were not significant. The authors concluded that ghrelin is sensitive to change in substrate oxidation. Jürimäe et al. [100] conducted a cross-sectional study to compare the resting total ghrelin levels of physically active and physically inactive adolescent girls. Accounting for age, body composition levels and pubertal stage, the investigators found lower plasma ghrelin levels in girls that had higher levels of body fat and that physically active girls had higher plasma concentrations of total ghrelin. Moreover, they reported that IGF-I was strongly related to ghrelin levels, a finding that the present authors reported earlier in this review in adults. Another cross-sectional study to determine relationship between physical activity (fitness) and total ghrelin measured over 24 h in 72 girls [101] revealed a positive relationship between total ghrelin and exercise frequency. Total ghrelin was also related to 24-hour LH concentrations in the postpubertal adolescent girls.

In summary, these data sets suggest that acute exercise does not typically increase total ghrelin concentrations. Moreover, they reveal that exercise training increases total ghrelin levels in adolescents and that ghrelin is sensitive to reductions in body fat or increases in energy expenditure in adolescents. These findings are similar to those in adults. Moreover, there is evidence that LH is a predictor of total ghrelin levels in girls and suggests that ghrelin is a biomarker of energy imbalance across the menstrual cycle [101].

Suggestions for Future Research

Although numerous studies have examined the effects of exercise on leptin levels in adolescents, more studies are needed to determine the discrepant findings to allow a better understanding of leptin changes in response to graded exercise. These investigations should examine changes in leptin with regard to caloric balance. There are no studies examining the effects of acute or chronic exercise on HMW adiponectin in adolescents and more studies using vigorous exercise protocols should be conducted to determine whether acute changes in adiponectin levels occur in adolescents. Whether body fat affects acylated ghrelin responses to exercise and whether training that reduces body composition affects acylated ghrelin requires further investigation.

References

1 Zhang Y, Proenca R, Maffei M, Barone M, Leopold L, Friedman JM: Positional cloning of the mouse obese gene and its human homologue. Nature 1994; 372:425–432.

2 Kraemer RR, Chu H, Castracane VD: Leptin and exercise. Exp Biol Med (Maywood) 2002;227:701–708.

3 Wake M: Issues in obesity monitoring, screening and subsequent treatment. Curr Opin Pediatr 2009; 21:811–816.

4 Lanigan J, Singhal A: Early nutrition and long-term health: a practical approach. Proc Nutr Soc 2009; 24:1–8.

5 Mostyn A, Symonds ME: Early programming of adipose tissue function: a large-animal perspective. Proc Nutr Soc 2009;68:393–400.

6 Jimenez-Pavon D, Kelly J, Reilly JJ: Associations between objectively measured habitual physical activity and adiposity in children and adolescents: systematic review. Int J Pediatr Obes. 2009;26:1–16.

7 Kim Y, Lee S: Physical activity and abdominal obesity in youth. Appl Physiol Nutr Metab 2009;34:571–581.

8 Fulton JE, Dai S, Steffen LM, Grunbaum JA, Shah SM, Labarthe DR: Physical activity, energy intake, sedentary behavior, and adiposity in youth. Am J Prev Med 2009;37(1 suppl):S40–S49.

9 Kraemer RR, Castracane VD: Exercise and humoral mediators of peripheral energy balance: ghrelin and adiponectin. Exp Biol Med (Maywood) 2007;232: 184–194.

10 Coleman DL, Hummel KP: Effects of parabiosis of normal with genetically diabetic mice. Am J Physiol 1969;217:1298–1304.

11 Crown A, Clifton DK, Steiner RA: Neuropeptide signaling in the integration of metabolism and reproduction. Neuroendocrinology 2007;86:175–182.

12 Castracane VD, Kraemer RR, Franken MA, Kraemer GR, Gimpel T: Serum leptin concentration in women: effect of age, obesity, and estrogen administration. Fertil Steril 1998;70:472–477.

13 Ahima RS, Flier JS: Adipose tissue as an endocrine organ. Trends Endocrinol Metab 2000;11:327–332.

14 Rosenbaum M, Leibel RL: Clinical review 107:Role of gonadal steroids in the sexual dimorphisms in body composition and circulating concentrations of leptin. J Clin Endocrinol Metab 1999;84:1784–1789.

15 Garcia-Mayor RV, Andrade MA, Rios M, Lage M, Dieguez C, Casanueva FF: Serum leptin levels in normal children: relationship to age, gender, body mass index, pituitary-gonadal hormones, and pubertal stage. J Clin Endocrinol Metab 1997;82:2849–2855.

16 Sih R, Morley JE, Kaiser FE, Perry HM 3rd, Patrick P, Ross C: Testosterone replacement in older hypogonadal men: a 12-month randomized controlled trial. J Clin Endocrinol Metab 1997;82:1661–1667.

17 Kapoor D, Clarke S, Stanworth R, Channer KS, Jones TH: The effect of testosterone replacement therapy on adipocytokines and C-reactive protein in hypogonadal men with type 2 diabetes. Eur J Endocrinol 2007;156:595–602.

18 Castracane VD, Kraemer GR, Ogden BW, Kraemer RR: Interrelationships of serum estradiol, estrone, and estrone sulfate, adiposity, biochemical bone markers, and leptin in post-menopausal women. Maturitas 2006;53:217–225.

19 Friedman JM, Halaas JL: Leptin and the regulation of body weight in mammals. Nature 1998;395:763–770.

20 Gallardo N, Bonzón-Kulichenko E, Fernández-Agulló T, Moltó E, Gómez-Alonso S, Blanco P, Carrascosa JM, Ros M, Andrés A: Tissue-specific effects of central leptin on the expression of genes involved in lipid metabolism in liver and white adipose tissue. Endocrinology 2007;148:5604–5610.

21 Ozcan L, Ergin AS, Lu A, Chung J, Sarkar S, Nie D, Myers MG Jr, Ozcan U: Endoplasmic reticulum stress plays a central role in development of leptin resistance. Cell Metab 2009;79:35–51.

22 Jasik CB, Lustig RH: Adolescent obesity and puberty: the 'perfect storm'. Ann NY Acad Sci 2008;1135: 265–279.

23 Ahmed ML, Ong KK, Dunger DB: Childhood obesity and the timing of puberty. Trends Endocrinol Metab 2009;20:237–242.

24 Golden NH, Carlson JL: The pathophysiology of amenorrhea in the adolescent. Ann NY Acad Sci 2008;1135:163–178.

25 Hilton LK, Loucks AB: Low energy availability, not exercise stress, suppresses the diurnal rhythm of leptin in healthy young women. Am J Physiol Endocrinol Metab 2000;278:E43–E49.

26 Welt CK, Chan JL, Bullen J, Murphy R, Smith P, DePaoli AM, Karalis A, Mantzoros CS: Recombinant human leptin in women with hypothalamic amenorrhea. N Engl J Med 2004;351:987–997.

27 Kraemer RR, Johnson LG, Haltom R, Kraemer GR, Hebert EP, Gimpel T, Castracane VD: Serum leptin concentrations in response to acute exercise in postmenopausal women with and without hormone replacement therapy. Proc Soc Exp Biol Med 1999; 221:171–177.

28 Kraemer RR, Durand RJ, Acevedo EO, Johnson LG, Synovitz LB, Kraemer GR, Gimpel T, Castracane VD: Effects of high-intensity exercise on leptin and testosterone concentrations in well-trained males. Endocrine 2003;21:261–265.
29 Weltman A, Pritzlaff CJ, Wideman L, Considine RV, Fryburg DA, Gutgesell ME, Hartman ML, Veldhuis JD: Intensity of acute exercise does not affect serum leptin concentrations in young men. Med Sci Sports Exerc 2000;32:1556–1561.
30 Elias AN, Pandian MR, Wang L, Suarez E, James N, Wilson AF: Leptin and IGF-I levels in unconditioned male volunteers after short-term exercise. Psychoneuroendocrinology 2000;25:453–461.
31 Fisher JS, Van Pelt RE, Zinder O, Landt M, Kohrt WM: Acute exercise effect on postabsorptive serum leptin. J Appl Physiol 2001;91:680–686.
32 van Aggel-Leijssen DP, van Baak MA, Tenenbaum R, Campfield LA, Saris WH: Regulation of average 24h human plasma leptin level; the influence of exercise and physiological changes in energy balance. Int J Obes Relat Metab Disord 1999;23:151–158.
33 Kraemer RR, Kraemer GR, Acevedo EO, Hebert EP, Temple E, Bates M, Etie A, Haltom R, Quinn S, Castracane VD: Effects of aerobic exercise on serum leptin levels in obese women. Eur J Appl Physiol Occup Physiol 1999;80:154–158.
34 Halle M, Berg A, Garwers U, Grathwohl D, Knisel W, Keul J: Concurrent reductions of serum leptin and lipids during weight loss in obese men with type II diabetes. Am J Physiol 1999;277:E277–E282.
35 Kohrt WM, Landt M, Birge SJ Jr: Serum leptin levels are reduced in response to exercise training, but not hormone replacement therapy, in older women. J Clin Endocrinol Metab 1996;81:3980–3985.
36 Pérusse L, Collier G, Gagnon J, Leon AS, Rao DC, Skinner JS, Wilmore JH, Nadeau A, Zimmet PZ, Bouchard C. Acute and chronic effects of exercise on leptin levels in humans. J Appl Physiol 1997;83: 5–10.
37 Kraemer RR, Acevedo EO, Synovitz LB, Hebert EP, Gimpel T, Castracane VD: Leptin and steroid hormone responses to exercise in adolescent female runners over a 7-week season. Eur J Appl Physiol 2001;86:85–91.
38 Pomerants T, Tillmann V, Jürimäe J, Jürimäe T: Relationship between ghrelin and anthropometrical, body composition parameters and testosterone levels in boys at different stages of puberty. J Endocrinol Invest 2006;29:962–967.
39 Souza MS, Cardoso AL, Yasbek P Jr, Faintuch J: Aerobic endurance, energy expenditure, and serum leptin response in obese, sedentary, prepubertal children and adolescents participating in a short-term treadmill protocol. Nutrition 2004;20:900–904.
40 Elloumi M, Ben Ounis O, Makni E, Van Praagh E, Tabka Z, Lac G: Effect of individualized weight-loss programmes on adiponectin, leptin and resistin levels in obese adolescent boys. Acta Paediatr 2009;98: 1487–1493.
41 Kelly AS, Steinberger J, Olson TP, Dengel DR: In the absence of weight loss, exercise training does not improve adipokines or oxidative stress in overweight children. Metabolism 2007;56:1005–1009.
42 Díez JJ, Iglesias P: The role of the novel adipocyte-derived hormone adiponectin in human disease. Eur J Endocrinol 2003;148:293–300.
43 Berg AH, Combs TP, Scherer PE: ACRP30/adiponectin: an adipokine regulating glucose and lipid metabolism. Trends Endocrinol Metab 2002;13:84–89.
44 Lihn AS, Pedersen SB, Richelsen B: Adiponectin: action, regulation and association to insulin sensitivity. Obes Rev 2005;6:13–21.
45 Camera A, Hopps E, Caimi G: Metabolic syndrome: from insulin resistance to adipose tissue dysfunction. Minerva Med 2008;99:307–321.
46 Guerre-Millo M: Adiponectin: an update. Diabetes Metab 2008;34:12–18.
47 Yang B, Chen L, Qian Y, Triantafillou JA, McNulty JA, Carrick K, Clifton LG, Han B, Geske R, Strum J, Brown KK, Stimpson SA, Pahel G: Changes of skeletal muscle adiponectin content in diet-induced insulin resistant rats. Biochem Biophys Res Commun 2006;341:209–217.
48 Li W, Tonelli J, Kishore P, Owen R, Goodman E, Scherer PE, Hawkins M: Insulin-sensitizing effects of thiazolidinediones are not linked to adiponectin receptor expression in human fat or muscle. Am J Physiol Endocrinol Metab 2007;292:E1301–E1307.
49 Scherer PE, Williams S, Fogliano M, Baldini G, Lodish HF: A novel serum protein similar to C1q, produced exclusively in adipocytes. J Biol Chem 1995;10;270:26746–26749.
50 Pedersen BK, Ostrowski K, Rohde T, Bruunsgaard H: The cytokine response to strenuous exercise. Can J Physiol Pharmacol 1998;76:505–511.
51 Nadeau KJ, Zeitler PS, Bauer TA, Brown MS, Dorosz JL, Draznin B, Reusch JE, Regensteiner JG: Insulin resistance in adolescents with type 2 diabetes is associated with impaired exercise capacity. J Clin Endocrinol Metab 2009;94:3687–3695.
52 Scheett TP, Mills PJ, Ziegler MG, Stoppani J, Cooper DM: Effect of exercise on cytokines and growth mediators in prepubertal children. Pediatr Res 1999; 46:429–434.
53 Sloan RP, Shapiro PA, Demeersman RE, McKinley PS, Tracey KJ, Slavov I, Fang Y, Flood PD: Aerobic exercise attenuates inducible TNF production in humans. J Appl Physiol 2007;103:1007–1011.

54 Nagaya N, Kojima M, Uematsu M, Yamagishi M, Hosoda H, Oya H, Hayashi Y, Kangawa K: Hemodynamic and hormonal effects of human ghrelin in healthy volunteers. Am J Physiol Regul Integr Comp Physiol 2001;280:R1483–R1487.
55 Kraemer RR, Aboudehen KS, Carruth AK, Durand RT, Acevedo EO, Hebert EP, Johnson LG, Castracane VD: Adiponectin responses to continuous and progressively intense intermittent exercise. Med Sci Sports Exerc 2003;35:1320–1325.
56 Ferguson MA, White LJ, McCoy S, Kim HW, Petty T, Wilsey J: Plasma adiponectin response to acute exercise in healthy subjects. Eur J Appl Physiol 2004; 91:324–329.
57 Punyadeera C, Zorenc AH, Koopman R, McAinch AJ, Smit E, Manders R, Keizer HA, Cameron-Smith D, van Loon LJ: The effects of exercise and adipose tissue lipolysis on plasma adiponectin concentration and adiponectin receptor expression in human skeletal muscle. Eur J Endocrinol 2005;152:427–436.
58 Jürimäe J, Purge P, Jürimäe T: Adiponectin is altered after maximal exercise in highly trained male rowers. Eur J Appl Physiol 2005;93:502–505.
59 Numao S, Suzuki M, Matsuo T, Nomata Y, Nakata Y, Tanaka K: Effects of acute aerobic exercise on high-molecular-weight adiponectin. Med Sci Sports Exerc 2008;40:1271–1276.
60 Cali AM, De Oliveira AM, Kim H, Chen S, Reyes-Mugica M, Escalera S, Dziura J, Taksali SE, Kursawe R, Shaw M, Savoye M, Pierpont B, Constable RT, Caprio S: Glucose dysregulation and hepatic steatosis in obese adolescents: is there a link? Hepatology 2009;49:1896–1903.
61 Diabetes Research in Children Network (DirecNet) Study Group: Adiponectin and catecholamine concentrations during acute exercise in children with type 1 diabetes. Pediatr Diabetes 2008;9:221–227.
62 Carrel AL, McVean JJ, Clark RR, Peterson SE, Eickhoff JC, Allen DB: School-based exercise improves fitness, body composition, insulin sensitivity, and markers of inflammation in non-obese children. J Pediatr Endocrinol Metab 2009;22:409–415.
63 Elloumi M, Ben Ounis O, Makni E, Van Praagh E, Tabka Z, Lac G: Effect of individualized weight-loss programmes on adiponectin, leptin and resistin levels in obese adolescent boys. Acta Paediatr 2009;98:1487–1493.
64 Kim ES, Im JA, Kim KC, Park JH, Suh SH, Kang ES, Kim SH, Jekal Y, Lee CW, Yoon YJ, Lee HC, Jeon JY: Improved insulin sensitivity and adiponectin level after exercise training in obese Korean youth. Obesity (Silver Spring) 2007;15:3023–3030.
65 Park TG, Hong HR, Lee J, Kang HS: Lifestyle plus exercise intervention improves metabolic syndrome markers without change in adiponectin in obese girls. Ann Nutr Metab 2007;51:197–203.
66 Nassis GP, Papantakou K, Skenderi K, Triandafillopoulou M, Kavouras SA, Yannakoulia M, Chrousos GP, Sidossis LS: Aerobic exercise training improves insulin sensitivity without changes in body weight, body fat, adiponectin, and inflammatory markers in overweight and obese girls. Metabolism 2005;54:1472–1479.
67 Ben Ounis O, Elloumi M, Lac G, Makni E, Van Praagh E, Zouhal H, Tabka Z, Amri M: Aerobic exercise training improves insulin sensitivity without changes in body weight, body fat, adiponectin, and inflammatory markers in overweight and obese girls. Ann Endocrinol (Paris) 2009;70:235–241.
68 Kondo T, Kobayashi I, Murakami M: Effect of exercise on circulating adipokine levels in obese young women. Endocr J 2006;53:189–195.
69 Kojima M, Hosoda H, Date Y, Nakazato M, Matsuo H, Kangawa K: Ghrelin is a growth-hormone-releasing acylated peptide from stomach. Nature 1999;402:656–660.
70 Filigheddu N, Gnocchi VF, Coscia M, Cappelli M, Porporato PE, Taulli R, Traini S, Baldanzi G, Chianale F, Cutrupi S, Arnoletti E, Ghè C, Fubini A, Surico N, Sinigaglia F, Ponzetto C, Muccioli G, Crepaldi T, Graziani A: Ghrelin and des-acyl ghrelin promote differentiation and fusion of C2C12 skeletal muscle cells. Mol Biol Cell 2007;18:986–994.
71 Kojima M, Kangawa K: Ghrelin: from gene to physiological function. Results Probl Cell Differ 2010; 50:185–205.
72 Sato T, Fukue Y, Teranishi H, Yoshida Y, Kojima M: Molecular forms of hypothalamic ghrelin and its regulation by fasting and 2-deoxy-D-glucose administration. Endocrinology 2005;146:2510–2516.
73 Volante M, Fulcheri E, Allìa E, Cerrato M, Pucci A, Papotti M: Ghrelin expression in fetal, infant, and adult human lung. J Histochem Cytochem 2002;50: 1013–1021.
74 Iglesias MJ, Piñeiro R, Blanco M, Gallego R, Diéguez C, Gualillo O, González-Juanatey JR, Lago F: Growth hormone releasing peptide (ghrelin) is synthesized and secreted by cardiomyocytes. Cardiovasc Res 2004;62:481–488.
75 Sakata I, Tanaka T, Matsubara M, Yamazaki M, Tani S, Hayashi Y, Kangawa K, Sakai T: Postnatal changes in ghrelin mRNA expression and in ghrelin-producing cells in the rat stomach. J Endocrinol 2002; 174:463–471.

76 Date Y, Nakazato M, Hashiguchi S, Dezaki K, Mondal MS, Hosoda H, Kojima M, Kangawa K, Arima T, Matsuo H, Yada T, Matsukura S: Ghrelin is present in pancreatic alpha-cells of humans and rats and stimulates insulin secretion. Diabetes 2002;51:124–129.
77 Hosoda H, Kojima M, Matsuo H, Kangawa K: Ghrelin and des-acyl ghrelin: two major forms of rat ghrelin peptide in gastrointestinal tissue. Biochem Biophys Res Commun 2000;279:909–913.
78 Caminos JE, Gualillo O, Lago F, Otero M, Blanco M, Gallego R, Garcia-Caballero T, Goldring MB, Casanueva FF, Gomez-Reino JJ, Dieguez C: The endogenous growth hormone secretagogue (ghrelin) is synthesized and secreted by chondrocytes. Endocrinology 2005;146:1285–1292.
79 Dixit VD, Yang H, Cooper-Jenkins A, Giri BB, Patel K, Taub DD: Reduction of T cell-derived ghrelin enhances proinflammatory cytokine expression: implications for age-associated increases in inflammation. Blood 2009;113:5202–5205.
80 Shintani M, Ogawa Y, Ebihara K, Aizawa-Abe M, Miyanaga F, Takaya K, Hayashi T, Inoue G, Hosoda K, Kojima M, Kangawa K, Nakao K: Ghrelin, an endogenous growth hormone secretagogue, is a novel orexigenic peptide that antagonizes leptin action through the activation of hypothalamic neuropeptide Y/Y1 receptor pathway. Diabetes 2001;50:227–232.
81 Nakazato M, Murakami N, Date Y, Kojima M, Matsuo H, Kangawa K, Matsukura S: A role for ghrelin in the central regulation of feeding. Nature 2001;409:194–198.
82 Wren AM, Small CJ, Abbott CR, Dhillo WS, Seal LJ, Cohen MA, Batterham RL, Taheri S, Stanley SA, Ghatei MA, Bloom SR: Ghrelin causes hyperphagia and obesity in rats. Diabetes 2001;50:2540–2547.
83 Chen HY, Trumbauer ME, Chen AS, Weingarth DT, Adams JR, Frazier EG, Shen Z, Marsh DJ, Feighner SD, Guan XM, Ye Z, Nargund RP, Smith RG, Van der Ploeg LH, Howard AD, MacNeil DJ, Qian S: Orexigenic action of peripheral ghrelin is mediated by neuropeptide Y and agouti-related protein. Endocrinology 2004;145:2607–2612.
84 Cummings DE, Purnell JQ, Frayo RS, Schmidova K, Wisse BE, Weigle DS: A preprandial rise in plasma ghrelin levels suggests a role in meal initiation in humans. Diabetes 2001;50:1714–1719.
85 Avram AM, Jaffe CA, Symons KV, Barkan AL: Endogenous circulating ghrelin does not mediate growth hormone rhythmicity or response to fasting. J Clin Endocrinol Metab 2005;90:2982–2987.
86 Arvat E, Di Vito L, Broglio F, Papotti M, Muccioli G, Dieguez C, Casanueva FF, Deghenghi R, Camanni F, Ghigo E: Preliminary evidence that ghrelin, the natural GH secretagogue (GHS)-receptor ligand, strongly stimulates GH secretion in humans. Eur J Endocrinol Invest 2000;23:493–495.
87 Date Y, Murakami N, Kojima M, Kuroiwa T, Matsukura S, Kangawa K, Nakazato M: Central effects of a novel acylated peptide, ghrelin, on growth hormone release in rats. Biochem Biophys Res Commun 2000;275:477–480.
88 Kraemer RR, Durand RJ, Acevedo EO, Johnson LG, Kraemer GR, Hebert EP, Castracane VD: Rigorous running increases growth hormone and insulin-like growth factor-I without altering ghrelin. Exp Biol Med (Maywood) 2004;229:240–246.
89 Schmidt A, Maier C, Schaller G, Nowotny P, Bayerle-Eder M, Buranyi B, Luger A, Wolzt M: Acute exercise has no effect on ghrelin plasma concentrations. Horm Metab Res 2004;36:174–177.
90 Zoladz JA, Konturek SJ, Duda K, Majerczak J, Sliwowski Z, Grandys M, Bielanski W: Effect of moderate incremental exercise, performed in fed and fasted state on cardio-respiratory variables and leptin and ghrelin concentrations in young healthy men. J Physiol Pharmacol 2005;56:63–85.
91 Kraemer RR, Durand RJ, Hollander DB, Tryniecki JL, Hebert EP, Castracane VD: Ghrelin and other glucoregulatory hormone responses to eccentric and concentric muscle contractions. Endocrine 2004;24:93–98.
92 Broom DR, Stensel DJ, Bishop NC, Burns SF, Miyashita M: Exercise-induced suppression of acylated ghrelin in humans. J Appl Physiol 2007;102:2165–2171.
93 Broom DR, Batterham RL, King JA, Stensel DJ: Influence of resistance and aerobic exercise on hunger, circulating levels of acylated ghrelin, and peptide YY in healthy males. Am J Physiol Regul Integr Comp Physiol 2009;296:R29–R35.
94 Redman LM, Veldhuis JD, Rood J, Smith SR, Williamson D, Ravussin E: The effect of caloric restriction interventions on growth hormone secretion in non-obese men and women. Aging Cell 2010;9:32–39.
95 Leidy HJ, Gardner JK, Frye BR, Snook ML, Schuchert MK, Richard EL, Williams NI: Circulating ghrelin is sensitive to changes in body weight during a diet and exercise program in normal-weight young women. J Clin Endocrinol Metab 2004;89:2659–2664.
96 Morpurgo PS, Resnik M, Agosti F, Cappiello V, Sartorio A, Spada A: Ghrelin secretion in severely obese subjects before and after a 3-week integrated body mass reduction program. J Endocrinol Invest 2003;26:723–727.

97 Pomerants T, Tillmann V, Karelson K, Jürimäe J, Jürimäe T: Ghrelin response to acute aerobic exercise in boys at different stages of puberty. Horm Metab Res 2006;38:752–757.
98 Mackelvie KJ, Meneilly GS, Elahi D, Wong AC, Barr SI, Chanoine JP: Regulation of appetite in lean and obese adolescents after exercise: role of acylated and desacyl ghrelin. J Clin Endocrinol Metab 2007;92: 648–654.
99 Nitsche H, Nitsche M, Sudi K, Tschop M, Zotter H, Weinhand G, Froehlich-Reiterer E, Gallistl S, Pirker M, Borkenstein M: Ghrelin: an indicator for fat oxidation in obese children and adolescents during a weight reduction program. J Pediatr Endocrinol Metab 2007;20:719–723.
100 Jürimäe J, Cicchella A, Jürimäe T, Lätt E, Haljaste K, Purge P, Hamra J, von Duvillard SP: Regular physical activity influences plasma ghrelin concentration in adolescent girls. Med Sci Sports Exerc 2007;39: 1736–1741.
101 Kasa-Vubu JZ, Rosenthal A, Murdock EG, Welch KB: Impact of fatness, fitness, and ethnicity on the relationship of nocturnal ghrelin to 24-hour luteinizing hormone concentrations in adolescent girls. J Clin Endocrinol Metab 2007;92:3246–3252.

Dr. Robert R. Kraemer
Department of Kinesiology and Health Studies, SLU10845
Southeastern Louisiana University
Hammond, LA 70402 (USA)
Tel. +1 985 549 2132, E-Mail rkraemer@selu.edu

Author Index

Subject Index